HEALING FLOATERS AND DETACHMENTS NATURALLY

A SIMPLE GUIDE TO GETTING RID OF THOSE PESKY SPECKS THAT AFFECT YOUR VISION

MARC GROSSMAN, OD, LAc
MICHAEL EDSON, LAc

SQUAREONE
PUBLISHERS

The information and advice contained in this book are based upon the research and the personal and professional experiences of the author. They are not intended as a substitute for consulting with a healthcare professional. The publisher and author are not responsible for any adverse effects or consequences resulting from the use of any of the suggestions, preparations, or procedures discussed in this book. All matters pertaining to your physical health should be supervised by a healthcare professional. It is a sign of wisdom, not cowardice, to seek a second or third opinion.

Typesetting and cover design: Gary A. Rosenberg

Square One Publishers
An imprint of The Globe Pequot Publishing Group, Inc.
64 South Main Street
Essex, CT 06426
www.globepequot.com

Library of Congress Cataloging-in-Publication Data

Names: Grossman, Marc, author. | Edson, Michael, 1955 author.
Title: Healing floaters & detachments naturally / Marc Grossman, OD, LAc,
    Michael Edson, LAc.
Other titles: Healing floaters and detachments naturally
Description: [Garden City Park, NY] : Square One Publishers, [2024] |
    Includes bibliographical references and index.
Identifiers: LCCN 2023031672 (print) | LCCN 2023031673 (ebook) | ISBN
    9780757005305 (paperback) | ISBN 9780757055300 (ebook)
Subjects: LCSH: Vision disorders--Alternative treatment. |
    Eye--Diseases--Alternative treatment.
Classification: LCC RE51 .G76 2024 (print) | LCC RE51 (ebook) | DDC
    617.7--dc23/eng/20231114
LC record available at https://lccn.loc.gov/2023031672
LC ebook record available at https://lccn.loc.gov/2023031673

Contents

Preface

We wrote this book to show you that, while medication or surgery is sometimes necessary to address an eye problem such as floaters, you can take control of your own vision care through nutrition and lifestyle choices. Taking an approach that focuses on prevention and support, we sought to offer a guide to eye health that embraces the body's ability to heal itself.

We wanted to give you the power to make sensible, informed decisions to promote the health of your eyes through the use of not only Western medicine but also complementary and alternative methods such as nutritional supplementation and traditional Chinese medicine. Of course, we also wanted to highlight diet and lifestyle choices as critical parts of the discussion when it comes to your vision. We firmly believe that combining various forms of healing is the way to achieve better health and preserve your vision, and we knew we had to put them all in one book.

The goal of *Healing Floaters and Detachments Naturally* is to educate readers about their vision difficulties, explain prevention strategies in regard to floaters and detachments, and explore the ways in which people with these vision disorders may preserve healthy eyesight. If you notice any change in vision, please contact your eye doctor right away to rule out any eye pathology that may need to be addressed.

Introduction

Perhaps you have been told that there is nothing you can do to get rid of the tiny spots or squiggly lines that appear in your field of vision from time to time. The advice most people with floaters are commonly given is to learn to live with them. The fact is, however, there is something you can do.

This book is designed to clear up the potential causes and symptoms of floaters and detachments. It also describes a number of ways in which you may treat or prevent pesky floaters and detachments. The techniques offered in this book are based upon the wisdom and practice of both modern-day and ancient medicine. The methods provided in the following chapters will show you how to become an active participant in your own vision care.

This book is divided into four parts. Part One focuses on the many possible causes and treatments of floaters. Part Two examines both vitreous and retinal detachments. It looks at where they come from and how they can safely be treated. Part Three looks at the many drugs people take and their side effects, which may lead to floaters and many other visual problems. Part Four offers the Vision Diet, a diet designed to strengthen and protect your vision.

The world of healthcare is ever changing. Our concepts of what Western medicine should be have shifted over the past few decades. Today's public wants a more comprehensive, integrated approach from healthcare providers. Complementary, integrated healthcare is slowly replacing the idea of referring each symptom to a different specialist. We need to look at the whole person, including a person's dietary preferences, exercise regimen, activities, and relationships. We need to determine what might have created these vision problems in the first place. Hopefully, this book is a first step towards doing just that. If you notice any change in vision, please contact your eye doctor right away to rule out any eye pathology that may need to be addressed.

PART ONE

Floaters

■ WHAT ARE FLOATERS?

Floaters are an appropriate name for the small dark shapes that appear before our eyes as we age. These spots may look like squiggles, strands, or any of a hundred other shapes. Although they can be annoying, floaters are typically harmless. If you suddenly become aware of floaters, however, they may signal a vitreous tear or detachment, or a more serious condition such as a retinal tear or detachment, particularly if they are accompanied by bright flashes of light, in which case you should contact your eye doctor right away.

HOW ARE FLOATERS FORMED?

As we age two things begin to happen. First, the *vitreous,* a gel-like fluid that keeps the shape of the eyeball round, starts to liquefy or clump and shrink. This creates a pulling on the *retina,* which is a light-sensitive layer of photoreceptor cells known as rods and cones at the back of the eye that processes light and is responsible for both daytime and nighttime vision. Second, the protein-based connective tissue that forms the vitreous lining weakens and tiny pieces of this connective tissue may float freely in the vitreous liquid.

3

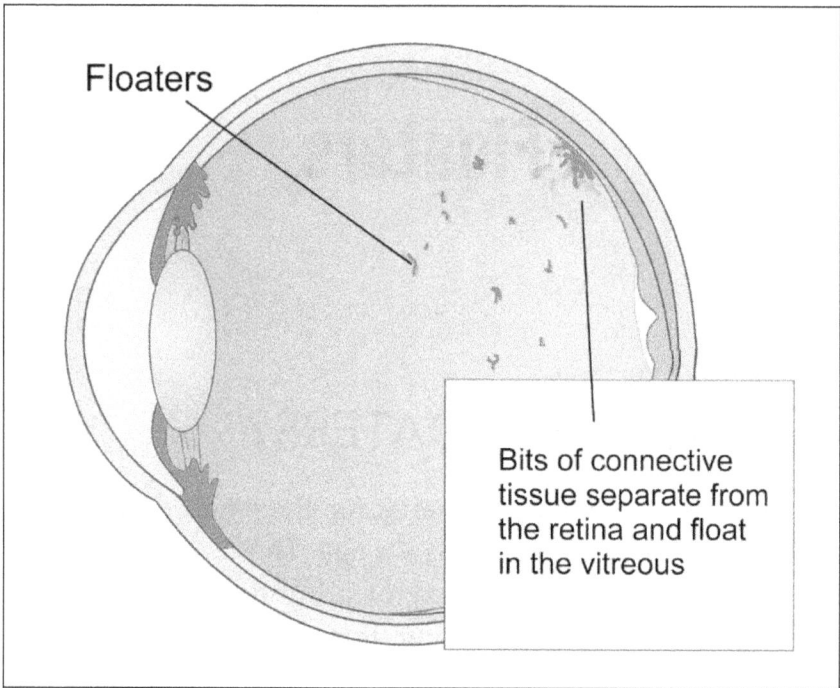

Floaters

Bits of connective tissue separate from the retina and float in the vitreous

Figure 1.1. Floaters

SIGNS AND SYMPTOMS

You know your own body better than anyone. Therefore, it is important to pay attention to the signals it sends you. Knowing the signs and symptoms of floaters will help you to know what is going on if you happen to experience any of the following:

- Visual spots that appear in the form of specks, strings, or clusters, or in any combination of these manifestations

- Movement of these visual spots when you move your eyes

- Drifting of these visual spots out of your line of vision when you do not move your eyes

As mentioned, a sudden appearance of floaters may indicate a retinal tear or detachment, or a vitreous tear or detachment. You should contact your eye doctor as soon as you can if you notice a significant number of floaters appear out of nowhere, particularly if these floaters are combined with flashes of light or a loss in vision.

RISK FACTORS

The vast majority of floaters are simply the result of changes in the eye that occur naturally as you get older. More than 50 percent of people over seventy years of age experience floaters. The technical term for the age-related breakdown of the eye's vitreous gel into liquid form, which allows pieces of connective tissue to float around this liquid, is called *vitreous syneresis*.[1]

Nevertheless, floaters have also been associated with a number of other risk factors, including:

* **Nearsightedness.** Those who are *nearsighted*—that is, those who have problems seeing things farther away—are more likely to develop eye floaters, particularly at a refraction of 6 diopters or over. (A *diopter* is a unit of measurement used to express the magnification strength of a lens.) Being born nearsighted means that the shape of the eye is more oval than round, resulting in chronic pulling on the retina, which over time can result in the weakening of the connective tissue between the vitreous and retina. The more nearsighted you are, the more oval the shape of your eye is. As you age, particularly after fifty years of age, a second risk factor appears, which is that the integrity of the vitreous starts to weaken, again resulting in additional stress on the connective tissue to the retina.[2]

The greater your level of nearsightedness, the higher your risk of experiencing vitreous tears and detachments (which often result in eye floaters), and the higher your risk of experiencing retinal tears and detachments (though vitreous tears and detachments are still more common).

- **Cataract surgery.** Patients often report floaters after cataract surgery, which are considered complications. One study that assessed different types of cataract surgery determined that patients whose eye surgeons used a surgical technique known as the *hinged capsulotomy* reported fewer floaters.[3]

- **Drug use.** The use of some prescription drugs or other drugs may cause floaters. Research has also found that certain topical drugs applied to the eyes may cause allergic reactions that can lead to floaters.[5]

- **Candidiasis.** People with *candidiasis,* a type of yeast infection, are at higher risk of developing floaters, perhaps due to an imbalance of flora in the gut that results in the body not being able to absorb nutrients properly and thus maintain eye health and integrity, similar to the possible effect of food allergies on the eyes.[7]

- **Hyaloid artery degradation.** Floaters may appear in babies during pregnancy as a result of a process known as hyaloid artery degradation. Prior to birth, the eyes of an unborn child contain an artery called the hyaloid artery, which regresses during the last three months of pregnancy. Sometimes, however, cell material is left behind and experienced as floaters. Pregnant mothers can take prenatal supplements to help support optimal development of the baby.[8]

- **Stress.** Chronic stress may contribute to the generation of floaters as well as other health conditions. Studies show that physical or emotional stress can lead to the onset of posterior vitreous detachment.[9] Developing a daily relaxation routine, such as meditation, can help you to relieve stress and improve your overall well-being immensely.

- **Inflammation.** Inflammation in the uvea or vitreous body can result in increased eye floaters.[10, 11]

- **Vitreous anomalies.** Retinal tears, leaky blood vessels, detachments, or other vitreous anomalies may be experienced as floaters. According to research, 11 percent of the population aged sixty-four to sixty-nine years old suffers from vitreous detachment, with the risk increasing with age.[12]

SIMILAR CONDITIONS

Some conditions may cause people to experience what seem like traditional floaters but are actually something a little different. Nevertheless, the frustration of seeing strange shapes appear in your field of vision out of the blue is the same.

- **Premacular bursa floaters.** Children and teens can experience a floater-like phenomenon that occurs within the *premacular bursa,* an area of liquified vitreous located in front of the macula. The *macula* is the central part of the retina where we get our most detailed vision. Although these "floaters" appear as a translucent web or spot on the eye, they are not real floaters, as they are not located within the vitreous. They are actually microscopic in size and appear large only because they are very close to the retina.

- **Blue field entopic phenomenon.** Also known as Scheerer's Phenomenon, this occurrence is defined by small bright dots appearing in the visual field and lasting for about a second. It is most often experienced when one is looking at the sky. These shapes are not technically floaters but rather white blood cells in the retina's capillaries, which cannot absorb the blue light and are therefore seen as bright dots.

■ CONVENTIONAL TREATMENT

There is no conventional treatment recommended for typical floaters. Patients are usually told they must learn to live with them. In more serious eye-floater conditions, vitrectomy surgery, a type of surgery used to treat problems of the retina and vitreous, may be recommended, although it risks the patient experiencing a number of side effects, including infection, increased pressure in the eye, excess bleeding, retinal detachment caused by the surgery, increased rate of cataract formation, and problems with eye movement. A few eye doctors in the United States have used laser treatment, but this procedure has not yet become a conventional option to address floaters.

■ COMPLEMENTARY AND ALTERNATIVE MEDICINE

Although there may not be any conventional treatments for floaters, there are a number of approaches in the field of complementary and alternative medicine, or CAM, which you might try to maintain eye health and thus avoid the problem. Certain supplements may help to prevent the onset of floaters, such as vitamin C, while research has shown that the body supplies the eye with nutrients that help support the vitreous gel and the connective tissue, such as hyaluronic acid.[13]

Used for thousands of years, *traditional Chinese medicine* (TCM) is based on the idea that illness results from the body's life force, or Qi, being out of balance. TCM states that Qi flows along pathways in the body known as *meridians,* which can become blocked or out of balance due to an imbalance of the opposing forces of yin and yang in the body. Meridian imbalances can be the result of different causes, including chronic stress, poor diet, lack of regular exercise or sleep, environmental exposure to toxins, and trauma. TCM seeks to restore balance to the body through the use of specific treatments, which include acupuncture and herbal remedies.

SUPPLEMENTS

Since floaters are often the result of vitreous tears or detachments, or clumping of the vitreous due to aging, supplements that support eye health may help to prevent them from occurring.

- **Vitamin C.** Vitamin C supports blood and lymph circulation, waste elimination, and connective tissue integrity. It is found in high concentrations in the eyes and helps to neutralize the effect of oxygenation in the ocular fluids.[14, 15, 16] As such, a daily vitamin C supplement (buffered and ascorbated) of 2,000 to 3,000 mg divided and taken with meals may be beneficial against floaters.

- **Hyaluronic acid.** Hyaluronic acid (hyaluronan) is a large molecule found in the vitreous gel that is believed to contribute to the vitreous' gel-like quality and possibly support the connective tissue located at the retina.[17, 18] As we age, the amount of hyaluronic acid in the body decreases, so a daily supplement of 100 to 200 mg is recommended.

- **Floater pellets.** Floater pellets contain a number of ingredients that are said to stimulate the body's natural ability to eliminate floaters. They are generally taken in doses of one to three pellets three times a day, preferably away from meals.

- **Glucosamine sulfate with MSM.** Glucosamine sulfate with MSM helps to build collagen and strengthen connective tissue.

- **Lutein.** Lutein is an essential nutrient for strengthening the retina.[19] A daily supplement of 6 to 20 mg may be helpful.

- **Zeaxanthin.** Zeaxanthin is an essential nutrient for strengthening the retina.[20] A daily supplement of 2 to 12 mg is recommended.

- **Omega-3 fatty acids.** Omega-3 fatty acids generally support retinal health, reducing the incidence and progression of retinal diseases.[21] A daily supplement of 2,000 to 3,000 mg is advised.

- **Multivitamin.** It may also be beneficial to take a whole-food multivitamin for the health of your body overall, including your eyes.

TRADITIONAL CHINESE MEDICINE

Traditional Chinese medicine views each patient as a unique person to be evaluated individually to determine the best treatment for a health issue. A TCM practitioner often looks at a patient's tongue and pulse and considers a number of other factors to ascertain the ways in which this person's meridians (energy pathways) are out of balance, and to decide the best way to treat this person to promote healing and reduce pain as quickly as possible.

Many of the main meridians run to the eyes. If one of these main meridians is not in balance, disease may result over time. The liver meridian, for example, runs from the big toe to the eyes, passing through the liver organ. A liver meridian imbalance can result is certain health and eye issues and may not be related to what is happening in the liver itself.

According to TCM, eye floaters can be related to a number of different imbalances in the body, including:

- poor circulation and storage of blood (often related to liver imbalances);

- poor absorption and distribution of essential nutrients (often related to spleen deficiency);

- poor production of blood (commonly related to kidney and spleen deficiencies); and

- congestion in the kidney, liver, and colon.

As the liver meridian is said to "open to the eyes," and is the primary energy pathway that supports healthy circulation, the free flow of energy in the eyes, and the free flow of energy throughout the body, common TCM therapies for floaters often address the liver meridian and include the following formulas:

- **Zhu jing wan** (preserve vistas pill) tonifies and nourishes the liver and kidneys, enriches the yin, and improves vision.

- **Ming mu di huang wan** (rehmannia pills to brighten the eyes) addresses problems related to liver blood deficiency, kidney yin deficiency, and liver yin deficiency.

- **Gui pi tang** (restore the spleen decoction) increases Qi, tonifies blood, strengthens the spleen, nourishes the heart, and helps the spleen to control the blood.

- **Xiao yao san** (rambling powder) is a classic liver tonic used in TCM.

TCM treatment strategies and herbal formulas recommended depend on a TCM practitioner's evaluation and can vary significantly.

■ LIFESTYLE CHANGES

In addition to TCM and supplementation, there are a few lifestyle changes that could help you to go a long way in strengthening your retinas and supporting the vitreous of your eyes.

- **Sunglasses.** Exposure to ultraviolet light, blue light from sunlight, and blue light from computer and television screens causes oxidative stress in the eye, affected the health of the eye. Invest in a good pair of sunglasses with ultraviolet protection on the lenses (100 percent UVA/UVB filtering), amber- or brown-colored polarized lenses are preferred. Wearing sunglasses whenever possible can be an important part of eye care, especially for older people, who typically suffer from weakened connective tissue between the retina and vitreous, with which vitreous detachments are associated.

- **Diet.** Foods that contain vitamin C, silica, MSM, or omega-3 fatty acids may help to maintain the integrity of the retina, vitreous, and connective tissue. Try to incorporate things like citrus fruit (vitamin C), green beans (silica), eggs or legumes (MSM), and cold-water fish such as salmon (omega-3 fatty acids) into your diet to boost your eye health.

- **Juicing.** Juicing can also help you to get the nutrients necessary for proper eye health. When making a juice, use your favorite fruits and vegetables, making sure to include four to six of the following: parsley, beets, carrots, celery, parsnips, apples, and raspberries. Be careful not to make it too sweet by using too many carrots or fruits. Try to use room temperature vegetables and fruit. Do not add ice or very cold liquids, as they would negatively impact the stomach's digestive juices. Do not juice as often during the cooler months of the year. Instead switch to vegetable soups or stews.

■ CONCLUSION

Eye floaters affect practically everyone as they get older, and because they are essentially harmless, it may seem as though you should simply accept them and move on. This attitude is likely reinforced by the fact that there is no conventional treatment for the problem. Nevertheless, you may not have to live with floaters forever. There are other approaches you may take to rid your life of this annoying phenomenon. Certain supplements, complementary and alternative therapies, and lifestyle changes may help to eliminate floaters directly, or they may boost your general eye health, which should help solve the issue indirectly.

PART TWO

Detachments

■ WHAT ARE DETACHMENTS?

Although posterior vitreous detachments and retinal detachments may seem like interchangeable conditions, they are not the same. Both eye problems often involve the appearance of floaters or flashes of light in the visual field, but a posterior vitreous detachment is not considered dangerous and does not threaten a person's eyesight. Its symptoms may fade over time, though the onset of eye floaters may cause a visual annoyance, depending on their size and location and the amount of light entering the eyes (floaters are more apparent, for example, at the beach). A retinal detachment, however, is an extremely serious issue and could lead to a loss of a person's eyesight. It typically requires major surgery to fix.

■ POSTERIOR VITREOUS DETACHMENT

Posterior vitreous detachment (PVD) affects 75 percent of people over the age of sixty-five, though it may be lessened in severity with dietary and nutritional changes. The prevalence of spontaneous PVD has been reported to be as high as 24 percent among patients aged fifty to fifty-nine years old, and

87 percent among patients aged eighty to eighty-nine years old.[22, 23] After occurring in one eye, PVD usually occurs in the other eye within six months to two years.[24]

In patients with symptoms of a PVD, there is an incidence of retinal tears of 14.5 percent, and hemorrhages of 22.7 percent. [25, 26] One study showed floaters in 42 percent, flashes in 18 percent, and both floaters and flashes in 20 percent of patients with PVD and secondary retinal pathology.[27] Only about 10 percent of patients with PVD develop a retinal tear. Around 40 percent of patients with an acute retinal tear, if left untreated, will develop a retinal detachment.[28] Therefore, it is crucial to get an immediate evaluation at the first appearance of symptoms.

A vitreous detachment is not sight-threatening and requires no medical treatment. In some cases of a partial vitreous tear, the remaining fibers can continue to pull on the retina, resulting in a macular hole, or potentially, a tear in the retina or retinal blood vessel. Again, this needs to be monitored by your eye doctor.

WHAT IS THE VITREOUS?

As described in Part One, the vitreous, or vitreous humor, is a gel that helps to maintain the integrity and structure of the eye. Taking up the space between the retina and the inner lens of the eye, the vitreous is composed of collagen fibers (about 0.5 percent), hyaluronic acid (about 0.5 percent), a small amount of ascorbic acid, and water (about 99 percent).[29, 30] As we get older, the vitreous becomes more liquid, and this causes a strain on the connective tissue and fibers between the vitreous humor and the retina, often resulting in a tear or detachment from the retina.

STRUCTURE

The vitreous humor fills the center of the eyeball, filling the space through which light passes between the lens of the eye and the retina at the back of the eye. Millions of fine fibers contained in the vitreous attach to the retina surface. There are no blood vessels in the vitreous. If a substance enters the vitreous humor, it will typically remain suspended in the gel. These substances can include blood, pieces of connective tissue, or clumps of cells, which are collectively referred to as floaters. Although 99 percent water, the vitreous does contain hyaluronic acid, hyalocytes that reprocess the hyaluronic acid, ascorbic acid, salts, sugars, vitrosin (a type of collagen), a network of collagen type II fibers, and a wide

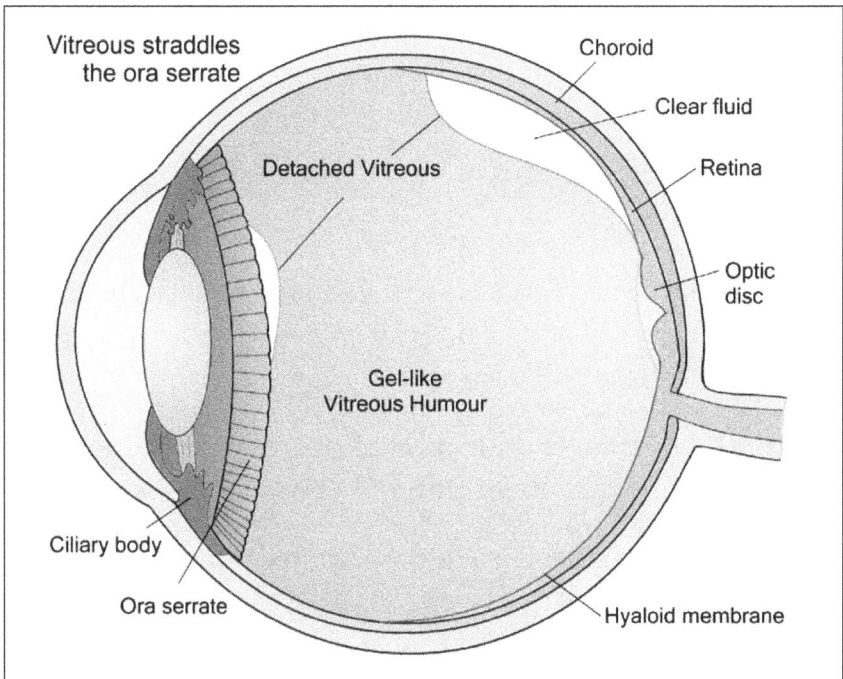

Figure 2.1. Vitreous Detachment

array of proteins in micronutrients. It also contains cells known as phagocytes, which remove waste cellular material over time.

A thin membrane of collagen called the *vitreous membrane,* or *hyaloid membrane,* encloses the vitreous. It is clear, transparent, and gelatinous (with two to four times the viscosity of water), and thins with age. Relatively speaking, the few cells it contains are mostly phagocytes.

The hyaloid membrane is attached only at the optic disc, where nerves pass from the photoreceptor system to the optic nerve, at the ora serrata, and on the top side of the lens, which is the junction of photosensitive and non-photosensitive areas of the retina. Vitrosin fibers floating within the vitreous are kept apart by electrical charges.

The most obvious purpose of the vitreous humor is to maintain a constant pressure, holding the shape of the eyeball in place.

TYPES OF POSTERIOR VITREOUS DETACHMENT

The pathology of PVD is always the same. Its effects, however, may be different. There is no way to predict exactly where a separation or tear will occur, but it may occur:

- at the ora serrata (the junction of the retina and the ciliary body), where the vitreous humor straddles it;

- at the optic disc, where the membrane is attached to the retina; or

- at a random place along the side of the hyaloid membrane (a thin transparent membrane enveloping the vitreous humor of the eye), leaving a space between the vitreous membrane and retina into which fluid can accumulate.

SIGNS AND SYMPTOMS

It is suggested that as much as 20 percent of PVDs are without symptoms.[31] While they do not usually cause any permanent vision loss, they can be annoying, particularly related to an influx of vitreous floaters. If you suspect you have a PVD, be on the lookout for symptoms such as:

- sudden detachment of the vitreous from the retina, often causing flashes that look like lightning or electric sparks;

- sudden change in the type, or an increase in number, of floaters; and

- sudden ring of floaters to the temporal side of vision (toward the ears).

These symptoms may last days or weeks, but it is critical to see your eye doctor at the first sign of any of them to rule out the possibility of a retinal tear or detachment, which is considered a medical emergency and a severe threat to vision. Your eye doctor will perform an immediate dilated retinal examination to determine whether you are dealing with a vitreous or retinal tear or detachment, or another condition altogether.

It is important to note that the risk of retinal detachment is greatest in the first six weeks following a vitreous detachment, but can occur over three months after the event. Between 8 and 26 percent of patients with acute PVD symptoms have a retinal tear at the time of the initial examination.[32]

RISK FACTORS

There are a number of different possible reasons for the occurrence of a posterior vitreous detachment, so if you are experiencing symptoms of PVD, you may want to consider if any of the following circumstances apply to you, as they may point to your actually having one.

- **Aging.** As the vitreous thins with age, the risk is greater.[33]

- **Nearsightedness.** People who are very nearsighted (more than 6 diopters) are at greater risk of vitreous and retinal tears and detachments.[34] Patients with nearsightedness, also known as *myopia*, experience PVD approximately ten years earlier than those with farsightedness, also known as *hyperopia*.[35, 36]

- **Cataract surgery.** This increases the risk for PVD. In one study, 75 percent of people with cataract surgery developed PVD.[37] This includes cataract surgery by phacoemulsification, which uses ultrasound to break up the lens, which is then removed manually and replaced with an artificial lens.[38]

- **Trauma.** Blows to the head, other trauma, and even vigorous nose blowing can cause vitreous detachments.

- **Computer use.** Excessive computer use may contribute to vitreous detachment, as it restricts the free flow of blood and energy to the eyes.

- **Menopause.** Menopause lowers levels of estrogen and hyaluronic acid, which may lead to changes in the vitreous. In premenopausal women, high levels of vitamin B_6 may be connected to more frequent PVD due to their estrogen-dampening effect.[39]

- **Drug use.** Injection of various intravitreal drugs, which are typically used for retinal bleeding in such disorders as wet macular degeneration, increase the risk of PVD.[40]

■ CONVENTIONAL TREATMENT

There is no specific treatment for posterior vitreous detachment, unless there is a retinal tear that needs to be surgically repaired. In more severe cases requiring a vitrectomy, there are several serious vision-threatening concerns that include bleeding into the vitreous humor, corneal edema, infection, elevated intraocular pressure (IOP), retinal detachment, and cataract formation. Thankfully, there are ways to strengthen the integrity of the vitreous and related connective tissue to the retina, which may help to prevent the condition from occurring.

■ COMPLEMENTARY AND ALTERNATIVE MEDICINE

Complementary and alternative therapies such as targeted supplementation, traditional Chinese medicine, and homeopathy may help to maintain a healthy retina and vitreous and prevent PVDs.

SUPPLEMENTS

For those that may be prone to vitreous tears or detachments, such as seniors, particularly if they are very nearsighted, targeted supplements can help keep the retina strong and healthy. If you decide to take supplements, we highly recommend regular checkups with your eye doctor to monitor your progress.

- **Lutein.** This carotenoid is well researched for retinal health and is essential in supporting the retinal pigment.[41] Research shows that taking lutein, zeaxanthin, and astaxanthin significantly improves visual acuity (vision sharpness).[42] The recommended daily dosage of lutein for retinal health is 6 to 20 mg.

- **Zeaxanthin.** Zeaxanthin is a potent antioxidant found in the retina that helps maintain the health of the retina.[43] A daily supplement of 2 to 12 mg should be taken with lutein.

- **Astaxanthin.** In a number of different studies, researchers found that astaxanthin was useful in reducing fatigue, dry eyes, and blurry vision, and recovery from intense visual stimulation.[44, 45] In computer users, astaxanthin was found to significantly improve *accommodation amplitude*, which refers to the ability of the eye to change focus as viewing distance changes. Studies also indicate that astaxanthin can be effective at ameliorating retinal injury.[46, 47]

- **Omega-3 fatty acids.** Half the retina is comprised of essential fatty acids. Research shows they have anti-inflammatory properties, which may be helpful against PVD.[48, 49] A supplement of 2,000 to 3,000 mg a day is recommended.

- **Hyaluronic acid.** Hyaluronic acid helps to strengthen connective tissue. It is found in the vitreous along with ascorbic acid, which is believed to support the integrity of the vitreous and related connective tissue to the retina.[50] A daily supplement of 100 to 200 mg is recommended.

- **Vitamin C (buffered and ascorbated).** Vitamin C helps to support the vitreous and connective tissue in the eye, and may react with oxygen in the ocular fluids.[51, 52] Depletion of ascorbate in the eyes reduces the ability of the vitreous to consume needed oxygen.[53] Supplementation with 2,000 to 3,000 mg of vitamin C a day, divided and taken with meals, is recommended.

- **Silica.** Silica helps to support connective tissue as well as bone health.[54] A daily supplement of 40 mg is recommended.

- **Bilberry.** Along with its ability to support night vision, bilberry is neuroprotective and has been shown to improve microcirculation.[55, 56, 57] A supplement of 120 to 180 mg is recommended.

- **Ginkgo biloba.** Ginkgo biloba contains many different flavonoids, including polyphenolic flavonoids, which have been proven to have antioxidative properties.[58] Numerous studies have shown that ginkgo biloba improves overall circulation, which helps the body to deliver essential nutrients and oxygen to the retina and eyes.[59] A supplement of 120 mg a day is recommended.

- **Vitamin D3.** Low levels of vitamin D are associated with retinal microvascular damage.[60] The most easily absorbed form of vitamin D is D3. Supplementation with 2,000 to 5,000 IU of Vitamin D3 a day may be beneficial.

- **Multivitamin.** A whole-food multivitamin can support your overall health, including the health of your eyes.

- **Proteolytic enzymes.** When taken between meals, proteolytic enzymes such as serrapeptase or nattokinase can help to break down debris in tissue and blood, and may help the body to break down floaters over time. Supplementation with 60,000 to 120,000 IU of serrapeptase in eight ounces of water, divided between meals, is recommended. The recommended dosage of nattokinase is 150 to 200 mg a day, taken between meals. (Larger dosages may be taken with your healthcare practitioner's guidance.)

TRADITIONAL CHINESE MEDICINE

In traditional Chinese medicine, the liver meridian "opens to the eyes" and is responsible for supporting overall eye health and the free flow of energy and blood to the eyes. So, for any eye issue, always consider liver support through both herbs and acupuncture.

The spleen and kidney meridians also help to nourish the eyes and support production of blood. From the perspective of traditional Chinese medicine, a common pattern to look for with PVD is "excess liver-gallbladder yang rising." In addition, since PVDs often occur as we age and are related to reduced circulation of essential nutrients, the formulas below may help to nourish and support these specific aspects.

- **Zhu jing wan** (preserve vistas pill) tonifies and nourishes the liver and kidneys, enriches the yin, and improves vision.

- **Ming mu di huang wan** (rehmannia pills to brighten the eyes) addresses problems related to liver blood deficiency, kidney yin deficiency, and liver yin deficiency.

- **Gui pi tang** (restore the spleen decoction) increases Qi, tonifies blood, strengthens the spleen, nourishes the heart, and helps the spleen to control the blood.

TCM treatment strategies and herbal formulas recommended depend on a TCM practitioner's evaluation and can vary significantly.

HOMEOPATHY

Homeopathy is an alternative form of medicine based on the belief that the body can cure itself. It uses small amounts of natural substances to stimulate the body's healing process. Homeopathic remedies are nontoxic medicines that are safe for everyone, including infants and pregnant or nursing women. Homeopathic remedies for PVD include the following preparations. You may use these remedies in 6X, 10X, 30X, 6C, or 30C potencies.

- #1 Calc fluor 6X for tissue integrity

- #2 Calc phos 6X for calcium strength

- #12 Silicea 6X to support connective tissue health

Cell salts may be useful against posterior vitreous detachments. Cell salt tablets are prepared in a homeopathic manner and typically contain twelve minerals, including forms of calcium, potassium, magnesium, sodium, iron, and silica. To make a cell salt solution, put up to ten tablets in a 16- to 24-ounce bottle, fill it with water, and swirl to dissolve tablets. Sip throughout the day.

■ LIFESTYLE CHANGES

In addition to TCM, supplementation, and homeopathy, there are a few lifestyle changes that could help you to go a long way in strengthening your retinas and supporting the vitreous of your eyes.

- **Diet.** Healthy eating programs like the Mediterranean diet or our Vision Diet (see page 55) can go a long way in preserving healthy vision and overall eye health. With these diets, it is important to avoid refined foods, that is, foods containing white flour, added sugars, or trans fatty acids, and fried foods. These include fast or processed foods. Keep overall sugar consumption low, and include healthy oils such as first cold-pressed extra-virgin olive oil in your diet. Consume plenty of fresh fruits and vegetables, and whenever possible, use organic products.

- **Juicing.** When making a juice, use some combination of the following ingredients: ginger, parsley, cabbage, beets, carrots, green leafy vegetables (such as spinach, kale, or Swiss chard), apples, celery, grapes, lemon, raspberries, wheatgrass, and chlorophyll. Do not use too much fruit, however, due to its high sugar content. (Berries, however, are lower in sugar than many other fruits.) It is best to use room-temperature vegetables and fruits, and not to add ice or cold liquids, since cold foods and liquids can negatively affect the stomach's digestive juices. Do not consume juices as often during the cooler months of the year. Instead switch to vegetable soups or stews.

■ RETINAL DETACHMENT

Retinal detachment (RD) is one of the most common causes for emergency room visits for critical eye issues. As explained in Part One, the retina is a thin layer of tissue in the back of the eye. When the retina detaches, it is lifted or pulled from its normal position. With a full detachment, the retinal cells are no longer being nourished by the blood. Total retinal detachment requires surgery for repair, and within twenty-four hours, or there will be permanent vision loss. Much like other eye-related issues that require immediate attention, including central retinal artery occlusion, chemical burns to the eye, and endophthalmitis (severe inflammation of the eyes, which is often due to bacterial or fungal infection), the sooner a person with RD can have surgery to repair it, the better. Approximately six to eighteen out of one hundred thousand people experience rhegmatogenous retinal detachment (see page 28) each year. Retinal detachment has a lifetime risk of 3 percent by age eighty-five.[61]

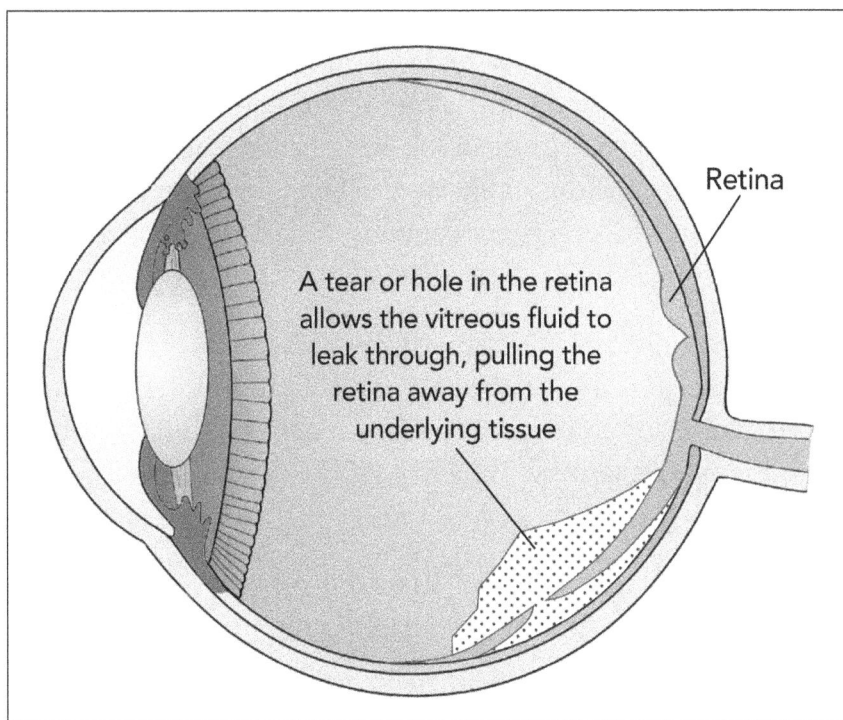

Retina

A tear or hole in the retina allows the vitreous fluid to leak through, pulling the retina away from the underlying tissue

Figure 2.2. Retinal Detachment

RETINAL LAYERS

The retina is made up of a number of layers, broadly divided by the inner neurons and photoreceptors and the outer retinal pigment epithelium (epithelium is a thin lining tissue); Bruch's membrane; and the choroid (fine blood vessels). The retina can detach when vitreous fluid within the eye leaks through a retinal tear, resulting in separation of the retina from its underlying tissue. The detachment may be small and not dangerous, or it could involve the entire retina, resulting in blindness if not treated quickly and properly.

TYPES OF RETINAL DETACHMENT

Retinal detachments may proceed unnoticed until a large section of the retina has detached. At this time, you may notice that part of your sight is missing (it could be vision loss from above, below, or off to one side). Sometimes patients say it as though a veil, curtain, or shade has been drawn on that part of the visual field. Types of retinal detachment include the following:

- **Rhegmatogenous.** *Rhegmatogenous retinal detachment* results from fluid leaking due to a tear or break in the retinal tissue. This issue causes the retina to separate from the retinal pigment epithelium, which provides it with blood and nutrients.

- **Tractional.** Less common than the others, *tractional retinal detachment* results from existing scar tissue in the retina causing stress on the retinal layers, which leads to a detachment from the retinal pigment epithelium. Existing scar tissue may be the result of chronic inflammation, past leakages, bleeding, etc.

- **Exudative**. *Exudative retinal detachment* results from fluid building up behind the retina without there being any tear in the retina, which eventually causes it to detach. It is often due to such eye conditions as wet macular degeneration, diabetic retinopathy, macula edema, or possibly eye trauma.

SIGNS AND SYMPTOMS

You know your own body better than anyone. Therefore, it is important to pay attention to the signals it sends to you. Knowing the signs and symptoms of retinal detachment will help you to know what is going on if you happen to experience the following:

- A sudden awareness of bright spots or streaks or dark moving specks, which may be floaters caused by the vitreous pulling on the retina.

- A sudden onset of blurred vision.

- Peripheral vision decreasing gradually or a curtain-like shadow over your vision.

Since a partial retinal detachment may or may not be dangerous, you should always see an eye doctor immediately after becoming aware of sudden bright spots or streaks, or experiencing a partial loss of vision.

RISK FACTORS

People who are nearsighted (also known as *myopic*) are at a greater risk for retinal tears and detachments due to the shape of their eyeballs being more oval than round. This causes more stress on the retina, including a potential thinning of the retinal wall. You are at higher risk of a retinal detachment if you:

- are severely nearsighted (greater than -6 diopters);

- have had an eye injury or cataract surgery;

- have a family history of retinal detachment;

- take glaucoma medications that decrease pupil size or cause eye muscle spasms;

- are over age fifty or have had age-related retinal tears;

- experience a blow to the head;

- have diabetic retinopathy or chronic eye infections that cause scarring; or

- have other eye disorders such as retinoschisis, uveitis, degenerative myopia, or lattice degeneration.

■ CONVENTIONAL TREATMENT

Retinal tears are typically treated with laser surgery, known as *photocoagulation*, or freezing, known as *cryopexy*, usually performed in a doctor's office. Full retinal detachments cause vision loss if not reattached within twenty-four hours. They usually involve in-hospital surgical repair in an operating room. For a partial retinal detachment, a procedure called *pneumatic retinopexy* may be recommended, in which the eye doctor injects a bubble of gas into the center part of the eye, known as the *vitreous cavity*. The head is positioned so that the bubble floats to the detached area and presses against the detachment. The eye doctor then uses a freezing probe or laser beam to seal the tear in the retina. The fluid that collected in the retina prior to this procedure then gets reabsorbed by the body.[62]

A surgeon may use silicone oil instead of gas when performing pneumatic retinopexy. While a gas bubble will dissolve in eye fluid over the course of a few days, silicone oil will not dissolve at all, instead requiring removal at a later date. This longer duration of effect can be beneficial in certain cases of retinal detachment.

In another common procedure called *scleral buckling*, doctors "indent" the sclera that is causing a ridge or buckle in the back of the eyes, reducing the pressure from the fluid underneath. This relieves some of the force caused by the vitreous tugging on the retina.

In a *vitrectomy*, the surgeon drains the vitreous fluid that maintains the shape of the back of the eye and replaces it with gas or silicone gel to help to flatten the retina and allow healing.

■ COMPLEMENTARY AND ALTERNATIVE MEDICINE

For people who are prone to retinal tears or otherwise more at risk of retinal detachments, supplementation and the use of traditional Chinese medicine may help to keep the retina strong and healthy. Regular checkups are highly recommended to monitor your progress as you use these methods.

SUPPLEMENTS

Targeted supplementation can encourage a healthy retina and vitreous, helping to prevent retinal tears and even improve recovery after surgery. The retina is replete with tiny blood vessels that provide the blood, nutrients, and oxygen necessary for a healthy retina and related tissue integrity. Supplements that support circulation to the retina can also help to reduce the risk of retinal detachment and keep vision strong.

- **Lutein.** Lutein is a strong antioxidant that is linked to the overall health and integrity of the retinal structure.[63] In an animal retinal-detachment model, lutein protected neuroreceptors in the eyes from cell death. It is a valuable adjunct to surgery for patients with retinal detachment.[64] A daily supplement of 6 to 20 mg may be helpful.

- **Zeaxanthin.** Along with lutein, zeaxanthin is a potent antioxidant found in the retina that helps maintain the health of the retina. A daily supplement of 2 to 12 mg is recommended.

- **Omega-3 fatty acids.** Essential fatty acids make up 50 percent of the retina. Supplementary or dietary fatty acids are essential for retinal health. Research also shows that they have anti-inflammatory properties.[65] Photoreceptor cells, which process light, require essential fatty acids to rebuild themselves, and a deficiency of DHA in the membranes of photoreceptors disturbs membrane fluidity and function, and can alter the process of outer segment renewal.[66] There is a deterioration of visual cells when DHA is deficient.[67] A daily supplement of 2,000 to 3,000 mg is advised.

- **Hyaluronic acid.** This nutrient helps to strengthen connective tissue and is found in the vitreous along with ascorbic acid (believed to help support the integrity of the vitreous and related connective tissue to the retina).[68] A daily supplement of 100 to 200 mg is recommended.

- **Vitamin C.** Vitamin C supports the vitreous and connective tissue. It is found in the vitreous gel and thought to encourage the integrity of the vitreous and related connective tissue to the retina, which we believe may reduce the risk of RD. A daily vitamin C supplement (buffered and ascorbated) of 2,000 to 3,000 mg divided and taken with meals may be beneficial.

- **Astaxanthin.** Astaxanthin is a potent antioxidant and a critical nutrient for eye support. It is able to cross the blood-eye barrier, supporting vascular health within the eye and protecting the eyes' photoreceptor cells.[69] Long-term damage to the retina due to sun exposure and free radicals weakens the retina and poses risks to healthy vision. A daily supplement of 6 to 12 mg is recommended.

- **Bilberry.** Along with supporting night vision, bilberry is neuroprotective and has been shown to improve microcirculation.[70, 71, 72, 73] A daily supplement of 120 to 180 mg is recommended.

- **Resveratrol.** Resveratrol may be protective against retinal detachment. Trans-resveratrol is a well-absorbed form of resveratrol. A daily supplement of 125 to 175 mg is recommended.

- **Grapeseed extract.** Grapeseed extract helps to strengthen blood vessels and reduce inflammation. A daily supplement of 200 mg is recommended.

- **Pycnogenol.** A daily supplement of 200 mg may have similar benefits to grapeseed extract.

- **Ginkgo biloba.** Ginkgo contains many different flavonoids, including polyphenolic flavonoids, which have been proven to exert antioxidative properties by delivering electrons to free radicals.[74] Numerous studies have shown that ginkgo biloba improves overall circulation.[75] A daily supplement of 120 mg is recommended.

- **Vitamin D_3.** Lower levels of vitamin D are associated with retinal microvascular damage.[76] The most easily absorbed form of vitamin D is D_3. A daily supplement of 2,000 to 5,000 IU of Vitamin D_3 is recommended.

- **Multivitamin.** It may also be beneficial to take a whole-food multivitamin for the health of your body overall, including your eyes.

TRADITIONAL CHINESE MEDICINE

The liver meridian supports a healthy flow of blood and energy to the eyes and throughout the body, while the spleen and kidney meridians support blood production and eye nourishment. An acupuncturist or herbalist will be best able to determine which herbal formulas are most relevant for supporting your eyes in regard to a weak retina, but here are some suggested eye formulas that can be helpful:

- **Zhu jing wan** (preserve vistas pill) tonifies and nourishes the liver and kidneys, enriches the yin, and improves vision.

- **Ming mu di huang wan** (rehmannia pills to brighten the eyes) addresses problems related to liver blood deficiency, kidney yin deficiency, and liver yin deficiency.

- **Gui pi tang** (restore the spleen decoction) increases Qi, tonifies blood, strengthens the spleen, nourishes the heart, and helps the spleen to control the blood.

EYE EXERCISES

As certain eye exercises may also be helpful against retinal detachment, daily practice of the following eye exercises is recommended:

Near and Far

This exercise is done to improve the flexibility of the eyes as they change from distance viewing to near visual focus.

To perform the near and far exercise:

- Take two deep breaths. (Remember to breathe regularly throughout.)

- Either sit or stand with your feet shoulder width apart. If you are standing, bend your knees slightly.

- Hold your thumb six inches away from your eyes and directly in front of your nose.

- Gaze easily at the thumb and take a deep breath. Then focus on a distant object at least ten feet away and take a deep breath. Change this focus every breath. Feel the muscles in your eyes change as you shift your focus.

Hot Dog

This exercise is done to improve the flexibility of the inside muscles of your eyes (called the ciliary muscles). It is important to keep those muscles flexible.

To perform the hot dog exercise:

- Take two deep breaths. (Remember to breathe regularly throughout.)

- Either stand or sit with your feet, shoulder width apart. If you are standing, make sure your knees are slightly bent.

- Focus on any target in the distance.

- While looking at your distant target, bring your index fingers, with the tips touching, about eight inches in front of your eyes and into your line of sight.

- Still aiming your eyes at the distant target, calmly notice a mini hot dog has appeared between the tips of your fingers. Remember to continue to breathe easily and deeply. Do not let the mini hot dog distract you and cause you to aim your eyes directly at it. Continue to aim your eyes toward the distant target.

- Pull the tips of your fingers apart slightly and observe the mini hot dog floating in the air.

- Keep the mini hot dog in your view for two breaths and then look directly at your fingers. The mini hot dog will disappear. Do not attempt to see the mini hot dog again for two breaths and then look in the distance and find it. Alternate between seeing and not seeing the mini hot dog for two minutes.

Scanning

Staring is bad for your eyes because it freezes your energy and muscles, restricting blood flow. Having your eyes scan things is the opposite of staring. Scanning objects in your environment keeps you alive and energetic.

To perform the scanning exercise:

- Take two deep breaths. (Remember to breathe regularly throughout.)

- Stand, sit, or move around your environment.

- As you look at objects, let your eyes glide over them as though you are painting them with your eyes. Continue to breathe deeply and easily.

- As your eyes shift from object to object, allow them to move easily without staring and continue breathing and blinking. They should move in a relaxed manner without any tension. Make sure to release any tension in the moth or the jaw.

ACUPRESSURE

Part of traditional Chinese medicine, the practice of *acupuncture/acupressure* is based on the belief that stimulation of specific areas on the skin known as *acupoints* can affect the functioning of different organs in the body, and that there exists currents of energy that flow in distinct patterns throughout the body called meridians. It is thought that when these currents of energy are flowing smoothly, there is health, but when any of these currents are blocked, there is pain and disease. Acupuncture uses needles to stimulate acupoints, while acupressure uses gentle fingertip pressure.

There are a number of acupuncture/acupressure points around the eyes (basically around the orbits of the eyes which are the bones that surround the eyeballs). The points shown below are some of the major local eye points.

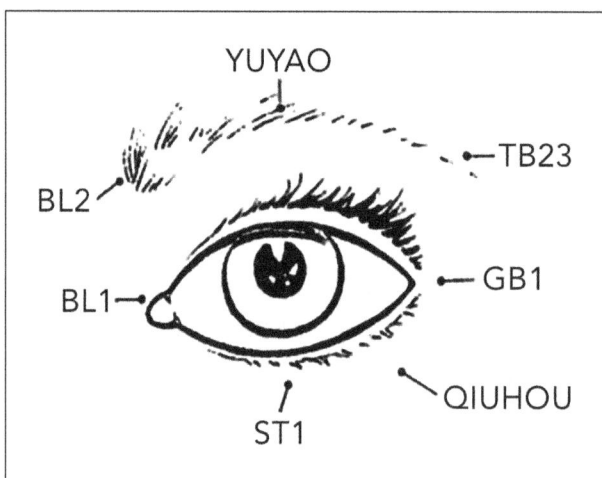

Figure 2.3. Major Acupressure Points

- **Jingming (BL1)** is a urinary bladder channel. It lies where the inner corner of the eye meets the nose. Bladder 1 and 2 are perhaps the best two points for eye problems of all kinds, from early-stage cataracts or glaucoma to hysteria with vision loss. They are also used for problems with conjunctivitis due to wind-heat or liver heat, and blurred vision in the elderly due to deficient jing and blood.

- **Zanzhu (BL2)** is a urinary bladder channel. It lies in the depressions at the inner ends of the eyebrows.

- **Yuyao** lies at the midpoint of the eyebrow in the hollow. It is good for eye problems related to worry, excessive study and mental strain.

- **Sizhukong (TB23)** is the San Jiao or triple burner channel. It lies in the depression at the outside end of the eyebrow. It is good for eye and facial problems, whether due to wind invasion or liver yang and fire.

- **Tongziliao (GB1)** is a gall bladder channel. It lies in the cavities on the outside corners of the eye sockets. It is good for eye problems such as conjunctivitis, red eyes, sore eyes, photophobia, dry eyes, itchy eyes, early-stage cataracts, and blurred vision, as well as for lateral headaches.

- **Qiuhou** lies midway between ST1 and GB1 along the orbit of the eyes.

- **Chengqi (ST1)** lies directly below the pupil on the infra-orbital ridge bone. It is a main point for all eye problems, including those due to wind cold, wind heat, and hyperactive liver yang.

Massage

To practice acupressure on yourself, gently massage each acupuncture point around the orbit of the eye, starting with BL1 and massaging each point as you go up and outward. Each point should be massaged for approximately five to ten seconds. You can massage both eyes at the same time. You can do this massage as often as you like over the course of the day. You may find that each point feels different in terms of sensitivity.

Breathe deeply and regularly as you perform the massage. Deep breathing helps the cells of your eyes to receive the oxygen they need to heal. Practice long, slow abdominal breathing while massaging the acupressure points.

If you are pregnant, consult a trained acupuncturist before treating yourself. Do not massage an area if it has a scar, burn, or infection.

Palming

Meant to reduce stress around the eye, *palming* is done without any glasses or contact lenses. By placing your palms around your eyes, you stimulate very powerful acupoints, helping to calm the mind, relax the muscles around the eyes, and bring healing energy to the eyes (through increased circulation).

To perform the palming exercise:

- Take two deep breaths. (Remember to breathe regularly throughout.)

- Sit in front of a flat table, lean forward, place your elbows on the table, and close your eyes gently.

- Place the palm of your left hand over your left eye, with your fingers on your forehead, and the hollow of your palm directly over the eye but not touching it. Allow room to blink. The heel of your hand should rest on the cheekbones.

- Place the other hand over the other eye, with your fingers crossing over the fingers of your other hand. The palm should be over the eye and the heel of the hand resting on the cheekbones.

- Make sure your elbows are low enough so that your face and the weight of your head are resting in your palms, being careful not to place any stress on your neck.

- Palming gives you the opportunity to focus on relaxing both your mind and your eyes simultaneously. Even though the suggested amount of time to engage in this therapeutic activity is approximately three minutes, palming can be done for as little or as much time as you like throughout the day as a way to relax your eyes, calm your mind, and let go of the tensions of daily life.

MICROCURRENT STIMULATION

Microcurrent stimulation (MCS) refers to the use of weak electrical signals to stimulate the muscles and skin. In relation to eye therapy with microcurrent stimulation, the process typically involves placing a damp cotton pad followed by a pad connected to an MCS device over each eye. The device is then switched on and runs a preprogrammed session, which generally lasts about five minutes. Standard recommended usage is four sessions of five minutes in length daily, or two sessions of ten minutes in length twice a day, totaling twenty minutes of microcurrent stimulation a day, although directions may vary based on circumstances.

When applied at home daily, microcurrent stimulation helps to support healthy circulation to the retina, increases energy production within the retinal cells, and helps the retina to eliminate waste. Daily MCS helps the body to get blood and nutrients to the retina, thus supporting healthy retinal tissue.

■ LIFESTYLE CHANGES

Since we consider most eye conditions to be a reflection of the health of the whole body, lifestyle choices that promote good health can play a major factor in getting and maintaining good vision.

- **Diet.** Studies show that patients can reduce their eye pressure by five to seven millimeters with an improved diet and supplement program. In general, a diet high in beta-carotene, vitamins C and E, and sulfur-bearing amino acids is recommended. Foods containing these nutrients include garlic, onions, beans, spinach, celery, turnips, yellow and orange vegetables, green leafy vegetables, seaweed, apples, oranges, and tomatoes. It is also important to drink lots of water, preferably eight to ten glasses of purified water daily. Avoid carbonated, caffeinated, and alcoholic beverages. They can actually dehydrate the eyes.

- **Juicing.** Juicing can also help you to get the nutrients necessary for proper eye health. When making a juice, use your favorite fruits and vegetables, making sure to include four to six of the following: parsley, beets, carrots, celery, parsnips, apples, and raspberries. Be careful not to make it too sweet by using too many carrots or fruits. Try to use room temperature vegetables and fruit. Do not add ice or very cold liquids, as they would negatively impact the stomach's digestive juices. Do not juice as often during cooler months of the year. Instead switch to vegetable soups or stews.

- **Exercise.** Do at least twenty minutes of aerobic exercise daily. Walking and swimming are two excellent forms of aerobic exercise.

- **Stress management.** It is important to manage your stress levels, which you may do by meditating, taking a walk in nature, practicing yoga or tai chi, using visualization techniques, praying, or engaging in some other practice that helps you to relax.

■ CONCLUSION

Every cell in your body is genetically engineered to try to heal your body as long as you are alive. Cells that cannot heal or become abnormal are targeted by the body for elimination, with new healthy cells created to replace them. As you age, your body will typically need more support than it did when you were young. Focused on the health of your vision, the recommendations in this part, which include dietary choices, supplementation, and the use of acupressure, can help you to maximize your body's healing potential, which is crucial in the fight against posterior vitreous detachment and retinal detachment.

PART THREE

Drugs and Their Side Effects

The human body is an organic unit with tissues and organs that are interrelated and mutually dependent. The health of the eyes can influence and be influenced by any other organ in the body. Prescription medications taken for all sorts of health problems can have visual side effects. Even herbs, foods, and vitamins can have side effects. Modern drugs are rapidly integrated throughout our bodies and can throw our systems out of balance. When prescribed properly, of course, drugs can help you to manage difficult health problems and even save your vision, so you must weigh the pros and cons with your physician before taking any medication.

Drug reactions are not always noticed immediately. Some medications produce gradual symptoms that eventually require a visit to a doctor. Sometimes this visit is to a doctor other than the doctor who prescribed the drug, and this second doctor may unknowingly prescribe one or more drugs to treat symptoms that are actually the side effects of the originally prescribed medication. To research the effects of drugs and their interactions, consult websites such as www.drugs.com, www.rxlist.com, and www.medscape.com.

Some drugs are associated with an increased risk of floaters as well as retinal and vitreous detachments. While you should always take your medication as directed, it is important to realize this connection if you have been prescribed one of these drugs and are at risk of floaters or detachments.

■ ANTIBIOTICS

Systemic antibiotics taken orally, intramuscularly, or intravenously to treat a bacterial infection may have eye-related side effects, including a higher risk of retinal disorders such as retinal detachments, which may result in trips to the emergency room.[74] Other eye problems associated with systemic antibiotic use include sensitivity to bright lights, dry eye syndrome, allergic conjunctivitis, temporary vision distortion (which can progress to night blindness), and increased risk of glaucoma (especially in patients who have diabetes).[75]

When antibiotics are given topically for eye problems, they may have side effects such as burning eyes or redness, pain, or swelling in or around the eyes. Certain types of antibiotics may cause puffiness or swelling of the eyelids or around the eyes, face, lips, or tongue; red, irritated eyes; yellow eyes or skin; increased sensitivity of skin to sunlight; allergic reactions; decreased visual acuity; pupil dilation, increased intraocular pressure; visual field defects; disturbances in color vision; double vision, or optic nerve damage.[76, 77, 78, 79, 80]

■ RETINAL BLEEDING MEDICATION

Lucentis, Avestin, and EyLea are the most common drugs taken by injection into the eyes to help stop bleeding in the retina and reduce inflammation. Ocular side effects from such injections may include conjunctival hemorrhage (up to 74 percent of users experience this side effect), eye pain (up to 35 percent), vitreous floaters (up to 27 percent), increased intraocular pressure (up to 24 percent), vitreous detachment (up to 21 percent), intraocular inflammation (up to 18 percent), visual disturbances or blurred vision (up to 18 percent), cataracts (up to 17 percent), foreign body sensation in eyes (up to 16 percent), eye irritation (up to 15 percent), increased lacrimation (up to 14 percent), blepharitis (up to 12 percent), dry eye (up to 12 percent), eye pruritus (up to 12 percent), ocular hyperemia (up to 11 percent), maculopathy (up to 11 percent), retinal disorder (10 percent), and possible higher risk of vitreous and retinal hemorrhage.

Less common side effects (affecting between 1 and 10 percent of patients) include retinal degeneration, retinal detachment or tear, retinal pigment epithelium break with or without detachment, reduced visual acuity, vitreous hemorrhage, vitreous disorder, uveitis, iritis, subcapsular cataracts, punctuate keratitis, corneal abrasion, anterior chamber flare, eye hemorrhage, conjunctivitis, allergic conjunctivitis, eye discharge, photopsia (light flashes), photophobia (light sensitivity), ocular discomfort, eyelid edema, eyelid pain, posterior capsule opacification, conjunctival hyperemia, endophthalmitis, and injection site hemorrhage.

Uncommon side effects (affecting between 0.1 and 10 percent of patients) include blindness, eye disorders of the anterior or outside parts of the eye (hypopyon, hyphema, keratopathy), iris adhesion, corneal deposits, corneal edema, corneal striae, injection site pain, injection site irritation, abnormal sensation in eye, and eyelid irritation.[82]

■ OTHER DRUGS WITH VISUAL SIDE EFFECTS

In addition to antibiotics and retinal bleeding medication, there are a number of other drugs that may have visual side effects, some of which are commonly used.

- **Acne drugs.** Many acne drugs are photosensitizing and can cause blurred vision, other changes in vision, excessive tears, eye discharge, or eye abnormalities, including microphthalmia.[83] Others may change the color of the white of the eye, reduce tear production, damage bilateral vision, or lead to sensations of dust in the eye, redness, burning eyes, temporary vision distortion, dry eye syndrome, or night blindness.[84]

- **Alzheimer's drugs.** Common ocular side effects of drugs for Alzheimer's disease include cataracts, eye irritation, and blurred vision. Less common side effects are dry eyes, glaucoma, blepharitis, retinal or conjunctival bleeding, spots before eyes, and periorbital edema.[85]

- **Antidepressants.** Antidepressants act on the nervous system change how information is processed in the brain. Any medication that affects neurological function can affect vision and cause changes in the cornea, optic nerve, lens, macula, or retina. Many antidepressants are drugs that increase your sensitivity to the sun and can make you more susceptible to cataracts, macular degeneration, double vision, conjunctivitis, dry eye syndrome, blepharitis, retinal hemorrhage, uveitis, and other eye problems.

- **Antihistamines**. Just as antihistamines have a drying effect on your nasal passages, they can also dry your eyes and contribute to cataracts, increased light sensitivity, burning and irritated eyes, and dry eye syndrome.[86, 87] In rare instances, they may make your pupils dilate or become unequal in size, decrease accommodation, increase blurred vision, or worsen narrow angles, which may induce angle-closure glaucoma.[88, 89] If you experience any unusual symptoms while taking an antihistamine, report them to your doctor.

- **Nasal steroids.** Long-term use of nasal steroids, commonly inhaled for asthma, is connected to open-angle glaucoma, as they can increase intraocular pressure. Newer nasal steroids are thought to have a minimal effect on intraocular pressure because of their low bioavailability.[90]

- **Birth control pills.** Women taking birth control pills have higher incidences of migraine headaches, problems with contact lenses due to dry eyes, color vision disturbances, corneal edema, lens opacities, retinal problems, and neuro-ophthalmologic complications.[91]

- **Blood thinners.** Blood thinners (also known as *oral anti-coagulants*), which are prescribed to prevent blood clotting, may cause blurred vision. Although rare, other side effects include swelling of the eyes or eyelids, yellow eyes and skin, and unusual bleeding or bruising.[92]

- **Cancer drugs.** Ocular side effects of cancer drugs can include blepharitis and eyelid dermatitis, excessive tearing, ocular irritation, conjunctivitis, keratitis, tearing, and blurred vision. In addition, tamoxifen, a *selective estrogen receptor modulator* (SERM), which is used to treat hormone-receptor positive breast cancer as well as osteoporosis, may cause posterior subcapsular cataracts, ocular pruritus, burning eyes, ocular pain, foreign body sensation in the eyes, or blurred vision. Make sure your ophthalmologist carefully monitors your eyes if you are undergoing cancer treatment.

- **Oral diabetes drugs.** Oral diabetes drugs can be photo-sensitizing. They absorb light energy and undergo a photochemical reaction, resulting in chemical modification of tissue. They can make you more vulnerable to cataracts, macular degeneration, macular edema, bladder cancer, and optic nerve degeneration, and can cause blurred vision and red, irritated eyes.[93, 94, 95, 96, 97]

- **Blood pressure medication.** Blood pressure drugs can cause the body to excrete excess fluid and ease the blood vessels. But in the eyes, less fluid can mean dry eyes, light sensitivity, blurred or double vision, dilated pupils, retinal hemorrhaging, or other changes or types of eye damage.[98, 99, 100, 101, 102]

- **Cholesterol-lowering drugs.** Cholesterol-lowering drugs may accelerate cataracts and cause fatigue, droopy eyelids, blurred vision, or eye irritation.[103,104] If you have high cholesterol, we suggest you add cholesterol-heathy foods to your diet, such as olive oil, oatmeal, soy, garlic, onions, shitake mushrooms, and red tice yeast, and supplement with vitamins C and E, niacin (vitamin B_3), and omega-3 fatty acids.

- **Benzodiazepines.** Prescribed for insomnia, these drugs may cause blepharospasm (eye twitch). Benzodiazepines can also lead to weaknesses in concentration and memory, as well as nystagmus, blurred vision, diplopia, pinpoint pupils, visual disturbance, difficulty focusing eyes, or cyclic movement of the eyelids.[105]

- **NSAIDs.** NSAIDs such as naproxen are popular drugs, available over the counter and in prescription strength. Side effects may include cataracts, dry eyes, or blurred vision.[106] Retinal hemorrhages might result from long-term use of these drugs. Unexplained diplopia and blurred vision mandate a detailed history of prescription painkiller use. Ocular side effects can infrequently include nonspecific visual distortions, minor hallucinations, and conjunctival yellowing.[107, 108]

- **Photosensitizing drugs.** Photosensitizing drugs, which include acne drugs and oral diabetes drugs, increase sensitivity to light. Use of these drugs may lead to eye problems, including cataracts and macular degeneration. Anytime you take a drug that makes you more sensitive to light, wear sunglasses that block 100 percent of ultraviolet rays, and take antioxidants such as vitamin C, vitamin E, vitamin A, selenium, alpha-lipoic acid, lutein, zeaxanthin, meso-zeaxanthin, and astaxanthin. When starting a new medication, ask your doctor whether it is photosensitizing.

- **Recreational drugs.** Recreational drugs have been shown to lead to retinal artery occlusion and rapid and often irreversible loss of vision, as well as decreased visual acuity, vasculitis, eye inflammatory conditions (episcleritis, panophthalmitis, endophthalmitis, scleritis), retinopathy, corneal ulceration, and transient visual losses.[109, 110]

- **Smoking tobacco.** Smoking significantly increases the risks of cataracts, age-related macular degeneration, diabetic retinopathy, open-angle glaucoma, retinal ischemia, anterior ischemic optic neuropathy, and Graves' ophthalmopathy. It is highly irritating to the conjunctiva and affects the eyes of nonsmokers through secondhand exposure. For pregnant women, cigarette smoke passes through the placenta, and the offspring of smoking mothers are prone to develop strabismus (a misalignment of the eyes).[111, 112]

- **Steroids.** Steroids are commonly prescribed for inflammatory conditions, including rheumatoid arthritis, lupus, Sjögren's syndrome, shingles, systemic poison ivy or poison oak, gout, and Crohn's disease. The most important ocular manifestations of which to be aware in steroid management are irreversible optic nerve damage in "steroid responders" (steroid glaucoma) and cataracts. Steroid use may cause ptosis, red eye, corneal deposits, and changes in color vision and the optic nerve. It may also damage the eyes indirectly by causing an increase in blood sugar, leading to diabetes.

  Steroid use can lead to blurred vision, cataracts (including posterior subcapsular cataracts), central serous chorioretinopathy, secondary bacterial infections (also fungal and viral), exophthalmos, glaucoma, or increased intraocular pressure.[113] Subcapsular cataracts will develop in up to fifty percent of people taking ten to fifteen milligrams of the steroid prednisone daily for one to two years. These cataracts are very dense and can cause a rapid loss of vision. They will not go away, even after you stop the medication, and will have to be surgically removed. If you must take a steroid, make sure you take high doses of antioxidants such as alpha-lipoic acid, vitamin C, vitamin E, and lutein to help prevent cataract formation.

  You can often identify a medication as a steroid by its name, which may end in "one" (e.g., prednisone, hydrocortisone, clocortolone) or "ide" (e.g., fluocinonide, budesonide, desonide), or include "pred" or "cort" (e.g., prednisolone, loteprednol, fluocortin).[114, 115, 116, 117]

■ ENVIRONMENTAL TOXINS

Prescription drugs are not the only chemicals that can negatively impact the health of your eyes. Many of the "safe" chemicals used in the home and yard are still toxic and can affect your vision directly or your overall health in general, thereby indirectly damaging your vision. Many herbicides and pesticides can harm your eyes and thus your vision.[118, 119, 120, 121, 122] Avoid the use of chemicals in the home, and herbicides and pesticides in the yard. If you have a food-producing garden, the avoidance of pesticides and herbicides is especially important.

■ CONCLUSION

When taken as prescribed, medications are important and sometimes essential. They can help to save and extend lives. But there can be side effects to taking prescription drugs, particularly in combination with other medications, and some of these side effects can result in vision changes. In light of this fact, be sure to review your medications and their potential side effects with your doctor and do your own online research on the subject as well.

PART FOUR

The Vision Diet

We believe that what we call the Vision Diet is a healthy diet for both the eyes and the entire body. It is a mainly plant-based diet, although it includes small portions of animal products (preferably organic, conscientiously produced animal products), such as meat (preferably from free-range, grass-fed animals). You may choose to follow a vegan diet, but be sure to check your levels of certain nutrients that are more difficult to obtain from plants, include vitamin B_{12} and iron, and supplement if any deficiencies arise.

In addition to being predominantly plant-based, the Vision Diet incorporates a few other principles, favoring certain foods and avoiding others.

■ ALKALIZE YOUR DIET

An alkalizing diet avoids foods that make your body more acidic, which often contribute to inflammation. Foods to limit or avoid include highly processed foods, refined carbohydrates, poor-quality oils, all types of sugar, and salt in excess amounts. A healthy diet, such as the Mediterranean diet, avoids overly processed or refined foods and is rich in vegetables and fruit, which are alkaline in nature and keep the body from having to counteract high levels of acidity—a fight that can deplete the body of much-needed minerals. Such a diet also provides a wide range of antioxidants, including those needed to support good vision and overall health.

■ BALANCE FATTY ACIDS

While both omega-3 fatty acids and omega-6 fatty acids are essential elements of a healthy diet, benefiting your heart, brain, eyes, circulation, metabolism, and even mental health, these two polyunsaturated fats are often out of balance in the body. Simply put, most people take in far too much omega-6s and far too little omega-3s. The recommended ratio of omega-3s to omega-6s is approximately 2:1 to 4:1, but the majority of individuals consume these fats at a ratio of about 15:1, which may lead to unwanted inflammation. (Not all omega-6 fatty acids are potentially inflammatory, however, such as those found in black currant seed oil, which actually has anti-inflammatory properties.)

Omega-3s and omega-6s are found together in many foods in various amounts. Omega-3s are found in high amounts in fish and other seafood, flaxseeds, chia seeds, and walnuts. Omega-6s are found in high amounts in corn, soybean, safflower, and canola oils, as well as eggs, tofu, walnuts, and almonds.

■ GO ORGANIC

Evidence is increasing that the nutritional value of fruits and vegetables is closely linked to the quality of the soil they are grown in. Evidence is also increasing that nonorganic foods are not the same as organically grown foods, as many conventionally grown foods contain residues of herbicides and pesticides.[123] Organic foods contain statistically higher levels of polyphenols, which are important for good health.[124] For example, organically grown tomatoes have seventy-nine percent more quercetin than nonorganic tomatoes, and organic tomato juice contains much more beta-carotene, rutin, flavonoids, and quercetin than nonorganic tomato juice. These differences may vary according to growing season. For example, the organic crop of a different season may have higher levels of vitamin C and quercetin.[125, 126]

A meta-analysis of research on organic compared with conventional dairy products found that the organic dairy products contained significantly higher amounts of protein, ALA, omega-3 and omega-6 fatty acids, and other nutrients.[127] Other research suggests that organic foods may be higher in vitamin C, iron, phosphorus, and magnesium, and many organic foods may have higher levels of anthocyanins, flavonoids, and carotenoids.[128]

Organic farming also delivers greater environmental benefits, making it the most sustainable farming method.[129, 130]

■ FAVOR THESE FOODS

The Vision Diet encourages the consumption of specific foods that are known to contribute to good health and may help to prevent eye problems such as floaters and detachments.

PURE WATER

Drink plenty of pure water every day, preferably spring water or filtered water. Nutritionists recommend drinking about half an ounce per pound of body weight daily, but you should drink what seems normal and natural. Water is essential for almost every cell activity. Being even slightly dehydrated reduces your metabolic efficiency. Chronic dehydration can lead to problems like kidney stones.[131] If you feel hungry much of the time, it might be that you are a little dehydrated. As a bonus, if you are trying to lose weight, drinking a glass of water before meals will help you feel full sooner.

Try to drink 1/4 cup of water at a time (when not exercising). This is the amount of water the kidneys easily absorb and process at one time. Excess water intake will stress the kidneys. In general, try to keep water near you and sip it from time to time.

It is important to note that tap water may include the following toxins: arsenic, aluminum, fluoride, pesticides, over-the-counter or prescription drugs, and disinfectant byproducts. Recommended home filters include reverse osmosis filters, ion exchange filters, and granular carbon or carbon block filters. If you use a filter that removes all minerals, such as a reverse osmosis filter, you should consider adding back the trace minerals with a mineral supplement in liquid form.

VEGETABLES AND FRUIT

The largest percentage of the diet should be made up of mostly vegetables and some fruit. Focus on eating dark leafy green vegetables and other colorful vegetables, as well as a few brightly colored fruits daily. These vegetables and fruits are rich in carotenoids, especially lutein and zeaxanthin, which are the pigments your eyes need to function well.

Carotenoids are pigments found in plants, in which they function as internal sunscreens, protecting the plants from solar radiation. Carotenoids are antioxidants that help to protect the body from oxidative damage. They are found throughout the body, but are highly concentrated in the eyes. When their levels in eye tissue are low, the risk of eye disease increases. For example, many studies report that the carotenoids found in vegetables significantly lower the risk of developing macular degeneration as well as diseases of the heart and brain.[132]

Even if you don't like green leafy vegetables such as collards, kale, and spinach, you can add them to soups, blend them into green drinks, or juice them with other fruits and vegetables. Aim to have 1/2 cup of cooked vegetables or one cup of uncooked vegetables at almost every meal.

WHOLE GRAINS

Whole grains supply protein, fiber, minerals, and some B vitamins (but not B_{12}). No single grain is healthier than any other.[133] Each grain supplies a unique blend of nutrients; therefore, enjoy a wide variety of whole grains. There is a good deal of debate as to whether organic and nonorganic grains are equivalent, but there has been evidence that the quality of the soil in which grains are grown makes a difference.

Whole grains are complex carbohydrates. They take a little longer to digest and help you maintain an even energy balance. They break down into glucose slowly. The slower the rate at which glucose is created, the more stable your blood sugar will be. Researchers report that whole grains, as opposed to processed (white or hulled) grains, can help you to stay healthy and ward off conditions such as high blood pressure and heart disease.[134] Proponents of food combining recommend that grains be eaten with healthy fats and vegetables. Grains are best digested in an alkaline environment.[135]

We recommend that you eat whole grains every day and vary your selection. Markets now offer a wide array of different types of grains. Try them all.

LEGUMES

Legumes are a great source of protein, carbohydrates, fiber, minerals, and vitamins, while being low in fat. They are also a good source of B vitamins (but not B$_{12}$) and contain antioxidant phytonutrients such as isoflavones and lignans. We recommend eating about $1/2$ cup of legumes at least two times a week, preferably served in the same meal with whole grains, as combining these two types of food will ensure your meal contains all the essential amino acids. While legumes are known to have high levels of phytates, which can hinder the body's absorption of nutrients, soaking legumes before cooking them reduces the amount of these compounds significantly.

HERBS AND SPICES

Try to substitute herbs and spices for salt or sugar as often as possible. They may contain many phytonutrients, including carotenoids and polyphenols. Use herbs and spices daily for all your meals. If you can, grow them fresh.

NUTS AND SEEDS

Nuts and seeds provide healthy fats, protein, vitamins, and minerals, including vitamin E, zinc, and essential fatty acids critical for retinal health. For example, pecans contain more than nineteen vitamins and minerals, and research has shown they may lower LDL cholesterol and promote healthy arteries.[136] Walnuts provide high amounts of anti-inflammatory omega-3 fats, along with high amounts of copper, manganese, molybdenum, and biotin. They also contain powerful free-radical scavenging antioxidants. Pistachios are high in lutein, beta-carotene, and gamma-tocopherol (vitamin E) compared with other nuts (all excellent nutrients for eye health). Almonds contain plenty of vitamin E, magnesium, and protein, and help to lower blood pressure and cholesterol levels, while also promoting weight loss and reducing hunger.

Sunflower seeds and other seeds are rich in vitamins and minerals, including vitamin E, copper, B vitamins, manganese, selenium, phosphorus, and magnesium, which support heart health and the immune system. Pumpkin seeds offer a wide variety of nutrients, including zinc, magnesium, manganese, copper, and protein.

We recommend eating a few nuts or seeds daily, and varying the kind of nut or seed for good balance.

OTHER SOURCES OF PROTEIN

For vegetarians, good sources of protein include fermented soy products, such as tempeh, which per ounce provides more protein than beef. For non-vegetarians, fatty fish, such as salmon (wild only), provide essential omega-3 fatty acids in addition to protein. It is important to note that smaller fish, such as herring and sardines, are lower on the food chain and tend to contain lower levels of heavy metals than larger fish, such as tuna.

∎ REDUCE THESE FOODS

A characteristic feature of most of the foods we suggest you limit or avoid is their ability to create inflammation in the body. Research shows that systemic inflammation is a contributing cause to eye disease and most chronic health conditions, including heart disease, diabetes, lung problems, and even emotional disorders.[137]

Certain foods increase oxidative stress in the body, which can lead to chronic inflammation. An overload of free radicals causes oxidative stress and plays a major role in the development of chronic and degenerative illnesses such as cancer, autoimmune disorders, rheumatoid arthritis, and neurodegenerative diseases. Oxidative stress is also implicated in age-related macular degeneration and cataracts.[138]

REFINED CARBOHYDRATES

Avoid or minimize refined carbohydrates in your diet, which are found in the white versions of bread, pasta, and rice. Most of the nutritional value of these foods is lost when their nutrient-rich husks are removed in processing. Furthermore, an abundance of these foods in the diet can lead to low levels of the enzymes and minerals needed to break down food properly. For those prone to chronic inflammatory conditions, these foods are quite acidic (as opposed to alkaline) and exacerbate body and eye inflammation.

Carbohydrates are sugar molecules and come in different forms. They are classified as simple or complex, depending on how quickly they are metabolized by the body. A simple carb, such as glucose, is absorbed very quickly, causing spikes in blood sugar. A complex carb, such as starch, is digested slowly—or, in the case of fiber, not digested at all—which also slows the absorption of simple sugars in food, thus preventing spikes in blood sugar. The glycemic index rates foods by how quickly they break down into sugar in the body. It ranks carbohydrates on a scale from 0 to 100, based on how quickly and how much they raise blood sugar levels after digestion.

A high glycemic index diet increases the risk of macular degeneration, diabetes, heart disease, and obesity.[139, 140, 141, 142, 143, 144, 145, 146, 147] A food with a glycemic index of 70 or above is considered high.[148] High glycemic index foods have an index of 70 to100 and include items such as white rice, white pasta, white bread, refined breakfast cereals, pretzels, French fries, couscous, millet, muesli, sugar-sweetened soft drinks, fruit juices, melons, pineapple, corn tortillas, sweet corn, and most salad dressings. Medium glycemic index foods have an index of 56 to 69 and include whole grain breads, rice cakes, oatmeal, brown rice, and whole grain pasta.

Research suggests that a low glycemic index diet has anti-inflammatory benefits.[149] Low glycemic index foods have an index of 55 or less. These foods include lentils, cashews, kidney beans, black beans, garbanzo beans (used to make hummus), oranges, apples, almonds, walnuts, peanuts (though these can be inflammatory and should be avoided for anyone with an inflammatory condition), carrots, bran cereals, all leafy greens, quinoa, millet, wild-caught fish, free-range beef, and eggs.

The glycemic index of a food can sometimes depend on certain factors. For example, the longer a starch is cooked, or the riper the fruit, the higher its glycemic index will be.[150]

SWEETENERS

Whether they get it from eating highly processed foods, candy, or soft drinks, Americans consume an enormous amount of sugar, the equivalent of more than seven tablespoons daily. This amount of sugar equals about 355 calories. We are in the midst of a crisis of obesity in the United States, and the consumption of sweet foods is part of the problem.

Sweeteners of all kinds contribute to inflammation. Sugar is one of the most acidic foods, and excess sugar in the diet is considered a leading contributor to illnesses such as type 2 diabetes, cardiovascular disease, high blood pressure (hypertension), dementia, and cancer.[151] Numerous research studies have linked many of these health conditions to eye diseases, including cataracts, glaucoma, and diabetic retinopathy. Studies have also linked diets high on the glycemic index with macular degeneration.[152, 153, 154]

When you eat or drink something sweet, it gives you a quick surge of energy. However, the consequence of glucose entering the bloodstream so quickly is that the body's ability to maintain equilibrium is compromised. With some attention to your diet, you can help to balance your blood sugar and overall system. This is especially true in the case of type 2 diabetes, which may be managed significantly through dietary choices.

High fructose corn syrup is one of the worst kinds of sweetener. It causes intracellular depletion of *adenosine triphosphate* (ATP), the primary compound that provides energy to the body. High fructose corn syrup also causes nucleotide turnover (these are the structural components of compounds such as DNA) and increases the generation of uric acid, which may have a critical role in causing diabetes and obesity.[155] There are a number of sweeteners that are chemically similar to high fructose corn syrup, which may be labeled as fructose, invert sugar, honey, evaporated cane juice, sugar, or sucrose.[156] Even when used in moderation, these sweeteners may contribute to cardiovascular disease, cancer, liver failure, and tooth decay.[157] They are also implicated in metabolic syndrome, memory problems, and many other health disorders.[158, 159]

Many people turn to artificial sweeteners to avoid sugar. One of the most popular artificial sweeteners is aspartame, which is found in many diet products. It is a synthetic chemical that when consumed breaks down into methanol, which may be converted into formaldehyde. Studies have linked aspartame to serious health problems, including neurological damage caused by toxicity to neurons in the brain and central nervous system.

Limit your sweets, avoid sugary drinks and sodas, and steer clear of foods that are high on the glycemic index. In general, an alkaline, anti-inflammatory diet will be a low-sugar diet. Avoid aspartame and other artificial sweeteners (typically found in foods labeled "diet").

FRIED FOODS

Fried foods provide almost no nutritional value and present digestive challenges. This is especially true of foods containing trans fats, which can cause diarrhea. Fried foods and foods containing trans fats substantially increase free radicals in the body, which cause the breakdown of healthy cells.

Excess intake of fried foods is tied to increased risks of diabetes and heart disease. One study found that people who ate fried food at least once per week had greater risks of type 2 diabetes and heart disease, and these risks increased as the frequency of fried food consumption increased. On a per-calorie basis, trans fats appear to increase the risk of chronic heart disease more than any other micronutrient.[160] In another study, participants who ate fried foods four to six times per week had a 39 percent increased risk of type 2 diabetes, and those who ate fried foods seven or more times per week had a 55 percent increased risk.[161]

The Dangers of Processed Foods

Breads, frozen meals, and other foods that have been created in "food factories" tend to be loaded with artificial sweeteners, flavor enhancers, and a host of preservatives. Many such chemicals have been gradually phased out as the food industry yields to scientific research proving their detrimental qualities. An example of this is the recent shift away from the use of certain food colorings.[162]

However, there are a number of food additives that have been banned in Europe but are still permitted for use in the US. These include but are not limited to Olestra, brominated vegetable oil, BHA/BHT, azodicarbonamide, rBGH or rBST hormones, and neonicotinoid pesticides.[163] Nevertheless, even when chemical additives are banned, new chemical additives are simply created as substitutes.

When you are at the grocery store about to buy prepared foods, look at the labels. If the food label includes any number of unidentifiable chemicals, you would be wise to avoid it or do some research before buying it. And if the first three ingredients include a refined grain, sweetener, or hydrogenated oil, it is best to pass it by.[164]

Cook from scratch whenever possible. Many healthy meals take no longer to prepare than frozen meals and are considerably better for you.

It is important to limit fried foods in your diet, especially deep fried foods. Avoid trans fats by staying away from hydrogenated products, such as shortening, which are made by combing liquid fat and hydrogen to make the fat solid at room temperature.

ADDITIVES

Processed foods all contain additives. These are ingredients that are designed to keep food from spoiling, supply an inexpensive source of flavor, or provide texture. They include phosphates, sulfites, and emulsifiers.[165]

- **Phosphates.** Many food additives contain phosphates, which increase danger for those with kidney disease and may contribute to heart disease, bone loss, and other chronic conditions.[166] These are often added as flavor enhancers. Phosphates that occur naturally in food are fine; the body absorbs them incompletely. However, added inorganic phosphates can significantly increase the blood phosphate level. The main problem is damage to the blood system, causing malfunctioning of the tissue that lines the blood vessels and accumulation of plaque.[167]

- **Sulfites.** When added as a preservative, sulfites break down vitamin B_1, especially under acidic conditions.[168]

- **Emulsifiers.** Emulsifiers help oil- and water-based liquids stay mixed together in foods. When you add a bit of mustard to your vinaigrette, you are adding an emulsifier. Early research reports that lab animals given chemical emulsifiers gained weight, had poor blood sugar control, and had more severe elimination problems. Artificial emulsifiers include gums, polysorbates 60 and 80, lecithin, and carboxymethylcellulose.[169]

Hidden Allergens

Potential allergens are hard to identify because they are undeclared, and they are the biggest cause of food recalls. Baked goods are the biggest source. The most common potential allergens are milk, wheat, soy, and sometimes nuts.[170] If you buy prepared foods, read the labels carefully, and avoid those with a long list of additives.

CAFFEINE

Caffeine may present challenges to the eyes. Caffeine is a stimulant found in cocoa beans, coffee beans, and black and green teas. Coffee, tea, and dark chocolate, however, have been found to have potential health benefits, too. For example, coffee contains antioxidant phenols, which may help to reduce the risks of developing neurodegenerative disease and other health conditions, including type 2 diabetes and liver disease. Thankfully, you can still get phenols from decaf coffee and tea, although some research suggests the amount would be slightly reduced.

On the negative side, coffee can increase serum homocysteine and cholesterol levels, and therefore may have adverse effects on the cardiovascular system.[171] In terms of eye health, one study showed that participants who reported drinking three cups or more of caffeinated coffee per day were at a higher risk of developing exfoliation glaucoma.[172] In contrast, another review of people who drink three to four cups of coffee a day (300 to 400 mg of caffeine) suggested that there is little evidence of health risk and some evidence of health benefits in association with cardiovascular disease, coronary heart disease, and stroke, when compared with those who did not drink coffee.[173, 174]

Traditional Chinese Medicine's Perspective on Coffee

Coffee is yang in nature. It regulates liver Qi (energy) and clears the gallbladder, resulting in its ability to protect against the formation of gallstones and alleviating constipation. Coffee moves Qi and blood, invigorates, and disperses (meaning that it has a diuretic effect and helps move energy and fluids in the body).

The benefits and risks of drinking coffee for eye and general health can depend on each person's constitution and the environment they live in. For people living in a cold environment, coffee can be very warming. For those living in a hot environment, it may create too much heat. Excessive amounts of coffee will agitate the liver yang. Symptoms can include headaches (typically on one side of the head or in or above the eyes), breaking blood vessels in the sclera, elevated eye pressure, red eyes, visual disturbances, ocular migraines, possible changes in eyesight, ringing in the ears, dizziness, dry mouth, heavy feeling, insomnia, and increases in blood pressure.

It can also stimulate internal wind, with symptoms that may include pain that moves around, itchy skin conditions, dizziness or vertigo, tremor or spasms, suddenly appearing rashes, sudden onset of headache or migraine with vertigo, or even sudden onset of disease. For people that are yang deficient (low in energy and generally cold overall), moderate amounts of coffee can be therapeutic to warm the body and stimulate yang. Excessive amounts can eventually have the opposite effect by depleting the adrenals.

In traditional Chinese medicine, food is divided into five natures: cold, cool, neutral, warm, and hot. Coffee brings warmth and heat to the body. So, a person who tends to have too much heat should avoid coffee or keep it at a minimum. Common symptoms of chronic heat include feeling hot, sweating all the time, being grumpy, having a swollen tongue, and often being constipated.

Coffee is also sweet and bitter. The slight sweetness of coffee also makes it mildly tonifying and nourishing. The primary bitter taste has the action of drying and dispersing. It can also clear heat, which helps to balance out the very warm nature of coffee. It reduces the risk of colon cancer as it moves Qi and blood in the large intestine.

Coffee can be helpful for those who tend to be cold or damp. Common symptoms of having a cold constitution include being pale, having cold hands and feet, sensitivity to cold temperatures, feeling weak, and having poor circulation. Dampness tendencies include being overweight (particularly around the stomach) dis-tended stomach, sticky mouth, greasy tongue, swelling, water retention, loose stools, and nodule masses (lymph nodes).

Try to limit yourself to one cup of coffee, tea, or cocoa daily, and have it unsweetened.

ALCOHOL

Alcohol reduces protective glutathione levels because it inter-feres with liver function. Although red wine has been touted for its antioxidant benefits, moderate consumption has been associated with an increased risk of breast cancer.[175] Heavy drinking increases the risk of many diseases, including heart disease, anemia, cirrhosis, depression, seizures, hypertension, immune system suppression, nerve damage, and pancreatic disease.[176]

Most alcoholics are malnourished, as the metabolism of alcohol by the liver prevents the proper digestion of proteins and vitamins. This is especially true in regard to vitamin A, which is essential for good vision. In addition, toxins and free radicals that interfere with fat digestion are created when alcohol is broken down in the liver.[177, 178]

Limit your alcohol consumption to one glass of red wine daily, if any.

■ CONCLUSION

The body needs proper nourishment to maintain good health and healing, particularly as you age. Focused on eating plenty of vegetables and fruit, and limiting or avoiding things like refined carbohydrates, sugar, trans fatty acids, and other unhealthy foods, the Vision Diet provides a guideline for supporting your long-term health and vision.

Conclusion

At the best of times, floaters are a nuisance. At the worst of times, they may signal a bigger problem such as a detachment. Maybe you have been dealing with tiny spots or squiggly lines appearing in your field of vision for years and thought there was nothing you could do about them. Now that you know the potential causes and symptoms of floaters and detachments, and the ways in which you may treat or prevent these conditions, you know better. You can become an active participant in your own vision care.

While you should be aware that certain drugs may have side effects that can lead to eye disorders, eye problems often end up being the result of a lack of essential nutrients being available to the eyes. The eyes need lifelong nourishment to maintain healthy vision and help to prevent eye disease. The chance of experiencing nutritional deficiencies increases as we age, often due to a number of reasons, which may include poor circulation, sedentary lifestyle, increased stress, poor diet, decreased ability to break down and absorb nutrients from food, or underlying health conditions. Most likely, however, it is within your power to counteract these factors of aging by fostering healthy habits. By making good choices in terms of your lifestyle and diet, as well as using appropriate complementary and alternative therapies when needed, you will strengthen and protect your vision and overall health. When you support your body, your body will support you—including your eyes.

Resources

To learn more about the natural approaches to vision problems and eye health mentioned in this book, you may wish to visit www.naturaleyecare.com. Based upon your specific eye disorder, the following organizations may also be able to provide you with information and help.

American Foundation for the Blind (AFB)
Website: https://afb.org
Phone: 214-352-7222

American Macular Degeneration Foundation
Website: www.macular.org
Phone: 888-622-8527

American Optometric Association
Website: www.aoa.org
Phone: 800-365-2219

BrightFocus Foundation
Website: www.brightfocus.org
Phone: 800-437-2423

Cambridge Institute for Better Vision
Website: https://bettervision.com
Phone: 978-768-3937

The Coalition for Usher Syndrome Research
Website: www.usher-syndrome.org
Phone: 855-998-7437

College of Optometrists in Vision Development (COVD)
Website: www.covd.org
Phone: 330-995-0718

Glaucoma Research Foundation
Website: https://glaucoma.org
Phone: 800-826-6693

Jack McGovern Coats Disease Foundation
Website: https://coatsdiseasefoundation.org
Phone: 888-314-8853

Lighthouse International
Website: https://lighthouseguild.org
Phone: 800-284-4422

MD Support
Website: https://mdsupport.org
Phone: 888-866-6148

National Eye Institute
Website: www.nei.nih.gov
Phone: 301-496-5248

National Keratoconus Foundation
Website: https://nkcf.org
Phone: 800-521-2524

Optometric Extension Program Foundation
Website: www.oepf.org
Phone: 410-561-3791

Prevent Blindness
Website: https://preventblindness.org
Phone: 800-331-2020

References

1. Gauger, E., Chin, E.K., Sohn, E.H. (2014). Vitreous Syneresis: An Impending Posterior Vitreous Detachment (PVD). Retrieved Jan 29 2018 from https://webeye.ophth.uiowa.edu/eyeforum/cases/196-PVD.htm.

2. Milston, R., Madigan, M.C., Sebag, J. (2016). Vitreous floaters: Etiology, diagnostics, and management. *Surv Ophthalmol*, Mar-Apr;61(2):211-27.

3. Alipour, F., Jabbarvand, M., Hashemian, H., Hosseini, S., Khodaparast, M. (2015). Hinged Capsulotomy – Does it Decrease Floaters After Yttrium Aluminum Garnet Laser Capsulotomy? *Middle East Afr J Ophthalmol*. Jul-Sep; 22(3): 352–355.

4. Haddrill, M., Diabetic Retinopathy. Retrieved Jan 29 2018 from http://www.allaboutvision.com/conditions/diabetic.htm.

5 Lyle, W.M., Hopkins, G.A. (1977). The unwanted ocular effects from topical ophthalmic drugs. Their occurrence, avoidance and reversal. *J Am Optom Assoc*. Dec;48(12):1519-23.

6. The interplay between gut bacteria and the yeast Candida albicans - PMC (nih.gov) https://www.ncbi.nlm.nih.gov/pmc/articles/PMC8489915.

7. Sallam. A., Lynn, W., McCluskey, P., Lightman, S. (2006). Endogenous Candida endophthalmitis. Expert Rev Anti Infect Ther, Aug; 4(4):675-85.

8. Oken, E., Bellinger, D.C. (2008). Fish consumption, methylmercury and child neurodevelopment. Curr Opin Pediatr, Apr; 20(2):178-83.

9. Flammer, J., Konieczka, K., Bruno, R.M., Virdis, A., Flammer, A.J., et al. (2013). The eye and the heart. *Eur Heart J*, May 1; 34(17): 1270-1278.

10. National Eye Institute. Facts About Uveitis. Retrieved Mar 29 2018 from https://nei.nih.gov/health/uveitis/uveitis.

11. Ibid. National Eye Institute. Facts About Uveitis.

12. Weber-Krause, B., Eckardt, C. (1997). Incidence of posterior vitreous detachment in the elderly. *Ophthalmologe*, Sept;94(9):619-23.

13. Stolyszewski, I., Niemcunowicz-Janica, A., Pepinski, W., Spolnicka, M. Zbiec, R., et al. (2007). Vitreous humour as a potential DNA source for postmortem human identification, Fola *Histochem Cytobiol*, 45(2):135-6.

14. Pirie, A. (1965). A light-catalysed reaction in the aqueous humor of the eye.

Nature, 205:500–501.

15. Takano, S., Ishiwata, S., Nakazawa, M., Mizugaki, M., Tamai, M. (1997). Determination of ascorbic acid in human vitreous humor by high-performance liquid chromatography with UV detection. *Curr Eye Res*, 16(6):589–594.

16. Eaton, J.W. (1991). Is the lens canned? *Free Radic Biol Med*, 11(2):207–213.

17. Brewton, R.G., Mayne, R. (1992). Mammalian vitreous humor contains networks of hyaluronan molecules: electron microscopic analysis using the hyaluronan-binding region (G1) of aggrecan and link protein. *Exp Cell Res*, Feb;198(2):237-49.

18. Jumper, J.M., Chang, D.F., Hoyt, C.S., Hall, J.L., Stern, R., et al. (1997). Aqueous hyaluronic acid concentration: comparison in pediatric and adult patients. *Curr Eye Res*, Oct;16(10):1069-71.

19. Piermarocchi, S., Saviano, S., Parisi, V., Tedeschi, M., Panozzo, G., et al. (2012). Carotenoids in Age-related Maculopathy Italian Study (CARMIS): twoyear results of a randomized study. *Eur J Ophthalmol*, Mar-Apr;22(2):216-25.

20. Richer, S.P., Stiles, W., Graham-Hoffman, K., Levin, M., Ruskin, D., et al. (2011). Randomized, double-blind, placebo-controlled study of zeaxanthin and visual function in patients with atrophic age-related macular degeneration: the Zeaxanthin and Visual Function Study (ZVF) FDA IND #78, 973. *Optometry*, Nov;82(11):667-680.e6.

21. Querques, G., Forte, R., Souied, E.H. (2011). Retina and Omega-3. *J Nutr Metab*, Oct 31:748361.

22. Hollands, H., Johnson, D., Brox, A.C., Almeida, D., Simel, D.L., et al. (2009). Acute-onset floaters and flashes: is this patient at risk for retinal detachment? *JAMA*, Nov 25; 302(20):2243-9.

23. Rahman, R., Ikramm K., Rosen, P.H., Cortina-Borja, M., Taylor, M.E. (2002). Ocular and systemic posaconazole(SCH-56592) treatment of invasive Fusarium solani keratitis and endophthalmitis. *Br J Ophthalmol*, Jul; 86(7):829.

24. Hikichi, T. (2007). Time course of posterior vitreous detachment in the second eye. *Curr Opin Ophthalmol*, May; 18(3):224-7.

25. Ibid. Coffee. (2007).

26. Dayan, M.R., Jayamanne, D.G., Andrews, R.M., Griffiths, P.G. (1996). Flashes and floaters as predictors of vitreoretinal pathology: is follow-up necessary for posterior vitreous detachment? *Eye (Lond)*,10 (Pt 4)():456-8.

27. Ibid. Dayan. (1996).

28. RNIB. Understanding posterior vitreous detachment. Retrieved Jan 14 2018 from tachment-pvd/posterior-vitreous-detachment-PVD.

29. Thimons, J.J. (1992). Posterior vitreous detachment. *Optom Clin*. 1992; 2(3):1-24.

30. Stolyszewski, I., Niemcunowicz-Janica, A., Pepinski, W., Spolnicka, M., Zbiec, R., et al. (2007). Vitreous humour as a potential DNA source for postmortem human identification, *Fola Histochem Cytobiol*, 45(2):135-6.

31. Richardson, P.S., Benson, M.T., Kirkby, G.R. (1999). The posterior vitreous detachment clinic: do new retinal breaks develop in the six weeks following an isolated symptomatic posterior vitreous detachment? *Eye (Lond)*, Apr; 13 (Pt2)():237-40.

32. Coffee, R.E., Westfall, A.C., Davis, G.H., et al. (2007). Symptomatic posterior vitreous detachment and the incidence of delayed retinal breaks: case series and meta-analysis. Am J Ophthalmol, 2007;144:409-13.

33. Foos, R.Y. (1972). Posterior vitreous detachment. *Trans Am Acad Ophthalmol Otolaryngol*, 76:480-497.

34. Gelia, L., Raman, R., Pal, S.S., Ganesan, S., Sharma, T. (2017). Incidence, Progression, and Associated Risk Factors of Posterior Vitreous Detachment in Type 2 Diabetes Mellitus: *Semin Ophthalmol*, 32(2):191-197.

35. Akiba, J. (1993). Prevalence of posterior vitreous detachment in high myopia. *Ophthalmology*, 1993 Sep;100(9):1384-8.

36. Wagle, A.M., Lim, W.Y., Yap, T.P., Neelam, K., Au Eong, K.G. (2011). Utility values associated with vitreous floaters. *Am J Ophthalmol*, Jul; 152(1):60-65. e1.

37. Ibid. Gelia. (2017).

38. Hilford, D., Hilford, M., Mathew, A., Polkinghome, P.J. (2009). Posterior vitreous detachment following cataract surgery. *Eye (Lond)*, Jun;23(6):1388-92.

39. Chuo, J.Y., Lee, T.Y.Y., Hollands, H., Morris, A.H., Reyes, R.C., et al. (2006). Risk Factors for Posterior Vitreous Detachment: A Case-Control Study. *Am J Ophthalmol*, 142(6):931-937.

40. Geck, J., Pustolla, N., Baraki, H., Atili, A., Feltgen, N., et al. (2013). Posterior vitreous detachment following intravitreal drug injection. *Graefes Arch Clin Exp Ophthalmol*, Jul; 251(7): 1691–1695.

41. Landrum, J.T., Bone, R.A., Joa, H., Kilburn, M.D., Moore, L.L., et al. (1997). A one year study of the macular pigment: the effect of 140 days of a lutein supplement. *Exp Eye Res*, Jul;65(1):57-62.

42. Piermarocchi, S., Saviano, S., Parisi, V., Tedeschi, M., Panozzo, G., et al. (2012). Carotenoids in Age-related Maculopathy Italian Study (CARMIS): twoyear results of a randomized study. *Eur J Ophthalmol*, Mar-Apr;22(2):216-25.

43. NIH. (2013). NIH Study provides clarity on supplements for protection against blinding eye disease. Retrieved Nov 10 2017 from https://nei.nih.gov/news/pressreleases/050513.

44. Astaxanthin (2002-2006) Reduces Eye Fatigue. Retrieved Nov 10 2017 from http://www.naturaleyecare.com/study.asp?s_num=272.

45. Nagaki, Y, Hayasaka, S, Yamada T, Hayasaka, Y, Sanada, M, et al. (2002). Effects of astaxanthin on accommodation, critical flicker fusions, and pattern evoked potential in visual display terminal workers. *J Trad Med*, 19(5):170-173.

46. Okazaki, Y., Okada, S., Toyokuni, S. (2017), Astaxanthin ameliorates ferric nitrilotriacetate-induced renal oxidative injury in rats. *J Clin Biochem Nutr*, Jul;61(1):18-24.

47. Ibid. Otsuka, (2013).

48. Udell, I.J., Abelson, M.B. (1983). Chemical mediators of inflammation. *Int Ophthalmol Clin*, 23:1:15-26.

49. Abelson, M.B., Butrus, S.I., Kliman, G.H., Larson, D.L., Corey, E.J., et al. (1987). Topical arachidonic acid: A model for screening anti-inflammatory agents. *J Ocul Pharmacol*, 3:63-75.

50. Ibid. Thimons. (1992).

51. Takano, S., Ishiwata, S., Nakazawa, M., Mizugaki, M., Tamai, M. (1997). Determination of ascorbic acid in human vitreous humor by high-performance

liquid chromatography with UV detection. *Curr Eye Res*, 16(6):589–594.

52. Eaton, J.W. (1991). Is the lens canned? *Free Radic Biol Med.* 11(2):207–213.

53. Shui, Y.B., Holekamp, N.M., Kramer, B.C., Crowley, J.R., Wilkins, M.A., et al. (2009). The Gel State of the Vitreous and Ascorbate-Dependent Oxygen Consumption. *Arch Ophthalmol*, Apr;127(4):475-482.

54. Jugdaohsingh, R. (2009). Silicon and Bone Health. *J Nutr Health Aging*, MarApr;11(2):99-110.

55. Matsunaga, N., Imai, S., Inokuchi, Y., Shimazawa, M., Yokota, S., et al. (2009). Bilberry and its main constituents have neuroprotective effects against retinal neuronal damage in vitro and in vivo. *Mol Nutr Food Res*, Jul;53(7):869-77.

56. Cohen-Boulakia, F., Valensi, P.E., Boulahdour, H., Lestrade, R. Dufour-Lamarinie, J.F., et al. (2000). In vivo sequential study of skeletal muscle capillary permeability in diabetic rats: effect of anthocyanosides. *Metabolism*, Jul;49(7):880-5. *NeuroToxicology*, 28 (2007) 93–100.

57. Zhu, Y., Xia, M., Yang, Y., Liu, F., Li, Z., et al. (2011). Purified anthocyanin supplementation improves endothelial function via NO-cGMP activation in hypercholesterolemic individuals. *Clin Chem*, Nov;57(11):1524-33.

58. Ou, H.C., Lee, W.J., Lee, I.T., Chiu, T.H., Tsai, K.L., et al. (2009). Ginkgo biloba extract attenuates oxLDL-induced oxidative functional damages in endothelial cells. *J Appl Physiol*, 2009;106:1674–85.

59. Chung, H.S., Harris, A., Kristinsson, J.K., Ciulla, T.A., Kagemann, C., Ritch, R. (1999). Ginkgo biloba extract

increases ocular blood flow velocity. *J Ocul Pharmacol Ther*, 15:233–40.

60. Mutlu, U., Ikram, M.A., Hofman, A., de Jong, P.T., Uitterlinden, A.G., et al. (2016). Vitamin D and retinal microvascular damage: The Rotterdam Study. *Medicine (Baltimore)*, Dec; 95(49): e5477.

61. Kang, H.K., Luff, A.J. (2008). Management of retinal detachment: a guide for non-ophthalmologists. *BMJ*, May 31;336(7655):1235-40.

62. Mayo Clinic. Retinal Detachment. Retrieved Mar 9 2018 from https://wwwsis-treatment/drc-20351348.

63. Jia, Y.P., Sun, L., Yu, H.S., Liang, L.P., Li, W., et al. (2017). The Pharmacological Effects of Lutein and Zeaxanthin on Visual Disorders and Cognition Diseases. *Molecules*, Apr 20;22(4)

64. Woo, T.T., Li, S.Y., Lai, W.W., Wong, D., Lo, A.C. (2013). Neuroprotective effects of lutein in a rat model of retinal detachment. *Graefes Arch Clin Exp Ophthalmol*, Jan;251(1):41-51.

65. Calder PC. (2003). N-3 polyunsaturated fatty acids and inflammation: from molecular biology to the clinic. *Lipids*, 38(4):343–352

66. Young, R.W. (1967). The renewal of photoreceptor cell outer segments. *J Cell Biol*, Apr; 33(1):61-72.

67. Santos, F.F., de Turco, E.B., Gordon, W.C., Peyman, G.A., Bazan, N.G. (1996). Alterations in rabbit retina lipid metabolism induced by detachment. Decreased incorporation of [3H]DHA into phospholipids. *Int Ophthalmol*, 19(3):149-59.

68. Thimons, J.J. (1992). Posterior vitreous detachment. *Optom Clin*, 2(3):1-24.

69. Goto, S., Kogure, K., Abe, K., Kimata, Y., Kitahama, K., et al. (2001).

Efficient radical trapping at the surface and inside the phospholipid membrane is responsible for highly potent antiperoxidative activity of the carotenoid astaxanthin. *Biochimica Biophysica Acta*, 1512:251-8.

70. Matsunaga, N., Imai, S., Inokuchi, Y., Shimazawa, M., Yokota, S., et al. (2009). Bilberry and its main constituents have neuroprotective effects against retinal neuronal damage in vitro and in vivo. *Mol Nutr Food Res*, Jul;53(7):869-77.

71. Yao, Y., Vieria, A. (2007). Protective activities of Vaccinium antioxidants with potential relevance to mitochondrial dysfunction and neurotoxicity. *Neurotoxicology*, 28 93–100.

72. Zhu, Y., Xia, M., Yang, Y., Liu, F., Li, Z., et al. (2011). Purified anthocyanin supplementation improves endothelial function via NO-cGMP activation in hypercholesterolemic individuals. *Clin Chem*, Nov;57(11):1524-33.

73. Cohen-Boulakia, F., Valensi, P.E., Boulahdour, H., Lestrade, R. Dufour-Lamarinie, J.F., et al. (2000). In vivo sequential study of skeletal muscle capillary permeability in diabetic rats: effect of anthocyanosides. *Metabolism*, Jul;49(7):880-5.

74. Ou, H.C., Lee, W.J., Lee. I.T., Chiu, T.H., Tsai, K.L., et a;/ (2009). Ginkgo biloba extract attenuates oxLDL-induced oxidative functional damages in endothelial cells. *J Appl Physiol*, 106:1674–85.

75. Chung, H.S., Harris, A., Kristinsson, J.K., Ciulla, T.A., Kagemann, C., et al. (1999). Ginkgo biloba extract increases ocular blood flow velocity. *J Ocul Pharmacol Ther*, 15:233–40.

76. Mutlu, U., Ikram, M.A., Hofman, A., de Jong, P.T., Uitterlinden, A.G., et al. (2016). Vitamin D and retinal microvascular damage: The Rotterdam Study. *Medicine (Baltimore)*, Dec; 95(49): e5477.

74. Etminan, M., Forooghian, F., Brophy, J.M. (2012). Oral Fluoroquinolones and the Risk of Retinal Detachment. *JAMA*, 307(13):1414-1419.

75. SWEye. How Antibiotics Can Damage Eyes and Vision. Retrieved Jun 14 2018 from https://eyes-and-vision.

76. RXList. Tetracycline. Retrieved Jun 8 2018 from https://www.rxlist.com/consumer_tetracycline_sumycin_actisite/drugs-condition.html.

77. Drugs. Amoxicillin Side Effects. Retrieved Jun 8 2018 from https://www.drugs.com/sfx/amoxicillin-side-effects.html.

78. Drugs. Tetracycline Side Effects. Retrieved Jun 8 2018 from https://www.drugs.com/sfx/tetracycline-side-effects.html.

79. Drugs. Amphotericin B Side Effects. Retrieved Jun 8 2018 from https://www.drugs.com/sfx/amphotericin-b-side-effects.html.

80. Gonzalez, S.N., Galvis, T., Borbolla, P., Mondragon, P., Juarz, O. (2017). Linezolid-associated optic neuropathy in a pediatric patient with mycobacterium nonchromogenicum: A case report. *Medicine (Baltimore)*, Dec;96(50):e9200.

82. Drugs. Lucentis Side Effects. Retrieved Jun 10 2018 from https://www.drugs.com/sfx/lucentis-side-effects.html.

83. RXList. Acutane. Retrieved Jun 2018 from https://drug.htm.

84. Stephenson, M. (2011). Systemic Drugs with Ocular Side Effects. *Rev Opthal-*

mol, Oct 4.

85. Drugs. Donepezil Side Effects. Retrieved Jun 10 2018 from https://www.drugs.com/sfx/donepezil-side-effects.html.

86. WebMD. Antihistamine Eye Drops. Retrieved Jun 8 2018 from https://tails.

87. Ibid. Jaanus. (1992).

88. Wren, V.Q. (2000). Ocular & Visual Side Effects of Systemic Drugs. *J Behav Optom*, 11;(6):149.

89. Caceres, V. (2016). Dermatology drugs, ocular side effects. *Eye World*, Sep.

90. Simsek, A., Bayraktar, C., Dogan, S., Karatas, M., Sarikaya, Y. (2016). The effect of long-term use of intranasal steroids on intraocular pressure. *Clin Ophthalmol*, 10:1079–1082.

91. Moschos, M.M., Nitoda, E. (2017). The impact of combined oral contraceptives on ocular tissues: a review of ocular effects. *Int J Ophthalmol*, 10(10): 1604–1610.

92. Drugs. Coumadin Side Effects. Retrieved Jun 8 2018 from https://www.drugs.com/sfx/coumadin-side-effects.html.

93. Lamb, T. (2011). Actos And Avandia Use Associated With Diabetic Macular Edema, Which Can Lead To Blindness. Retrieved Jun 7 2018 from fect-eye-disease-diabetic-macular-edema-dme-blindness.html.

94. Simo, R., Hernandez, C. (2017). GLP-1R as a Target for the Treatment of Diabetic Retinopathy: Friend or Foe? *Diabetes*, Jun;66(6):1453-1460.

95. Ibid. Lamb. (2011).

96. Miller, N.R. (2007). Optic Neuropathies. Retrieved June 8 2018 from https://www.sciencedirect.com/topics/neuroscience/optic-neuropathy.

97. Drugs. Chlorpropamide Side Effects. Retrieved June 9 2018 from https://www.drugs.com/sfx/chlorpropamide-side-effects.html.

98. Drugs. Lasix Side Effects. Retrieved June 9 2018 from https://www.drugs.com/sfx/lasix-side-effects.html.

99. Muchnick, B.G. (2013). Which Side Effects of Lurking in the Shadows? *Rev Optom*, Feb 15.

100. Petrounis AD, Akritopoulos P. (1989). Influence of topical and systemic beta-blockers on tear production. *Int Ophthalmol*, Jan;13(1-2):75-80.

101. Drugs. Clonidine Side Effects. Retrieved June 9 2018 from https://www.drugs.com/sfx/clonidine-side-effects.html.

102. Drugs. Catapres Side Effects. Retrieved June 9 2018 from https://www.rxlist.com/catapres-drug.htm#side_effects_interactions.

103. Fraundfelder FW, Fraunfelder FT, (2012). Drug-related adverse effects of clinical importance to the opthalmologist. Course presented at the American Academy of Opthalmology Annual Meeting, Chicago. November 10-13.

104. Mills, E.J., Wu, P., Chong, G., Ghement, I., Singh, S., et al. (2011). Efficacy and safety of statin treatment for cardiovascular disease: a network meta-analysis of 170,255 patients from 76 randomized trials. *QJM*, Feb;104(2):109-24.

105. Drugs. Midazolam Side Effects. Retrieved June 9 2018 from https://www.drugs.com/sfx/midazolam-side-effects.html.

106. Drugs. Naproxen Side Effects. Retrieved June 9 2018 from https://www.drugs.com/sfx/naproxen-side-effects.html.

107. Richa S, Yazbek J. (2010). Ocular adverse effects of common psychotropic agents: a review. *CNS drugs,* Jun;24(6):501-26.

108. Bookwalter T, Gitlin M. (2005). Gabapentin-induced neurologic toxicities. *Pharmacotherapy,* Dec;25(12):1817-9.

109. Mantelli, F., Lambiase, A., Sacchetti, M., Orlandi, V., Rosa, A., et al. (2015). Cocaine snorting may induce ocular surface damage through corneal sensitivity impairment. *Graefes Arch Clin Exp Ophthalmol,* May;253(5):765-72.

110. Hazin, R., Cadet, J.L., Kahook, M.Y., Saed, D. (2009). Ocular manifestations of crystal methamphetamine use. *Neurotox Res,* Feb;15(2):187-91.

111. Klein, B.E., Klein, R. (2007). Lifestyle exposures and eye diseases in adults.

Am J Ophthalmol, Dec; 144(6):961-969.

112. Solberg, Y., Rosner, M., Belkin, M. (1998). The association between cigarette smoking and ocular disease. *Surv Ophthalmol,* May-Jun;42(6):535-47.

113 Drugs. Prednisone Side Effects. Retrieved Jun 10 2018 from https://www.drugs.com/sfx/prednisone-side-effects.html.

114. Oto, B. (2011). Drug Families: Steroids and Antibiotics. Retrieved Jun 7 2018 from ics.

115. Ibid. Oto. (2011).

116. Ibid. Oto. (2011).

117. Ibid. Oto. (2011).

118. Seoane, A., Espejo, M., Pallas, M., Rodriguez-Farre, E., Ambrosio, S., et al. (1999). Degeneration and gliosis in rat retina and central nervous system from 3,3'-iminodipropionitrile exposure. *Brain Res,* Jul 3:833(2):258-71.

119. Roy, N.M., Carneiro, B., Ochs, J. (2016). Glyphosate induces neurotoxicity in zebrafish. *Environ Toxicol Pharmacol,* Mar;42:45-54.

120. Timchaulk, C., Dryzga, M.D., Johnson, K.A., Eddy, S.L., Freshour, N.L. (1997). Comparative pharmacokinetics of [14C] metosulam (N-[2,6-dichloro-3methylphenyl]-5,7-dimethoxy-1,2,4triazolo[1,5a]-pyrimidine-2-sulfonamide) in rats, mice and dogs. *J Appl Toxicol,* Jan-Feb; 17(1):9-21.

121. Kamal, M.A., Al-jafari, A.A. (1999). Kinetic constants for the inhibition of camel retinal acetylcholinesterase by the carbamate insecticide lanate. *J Biochem Mol Toxicol,* 1999;13(1):41-6.

122. Paganelli, A., Gnazzo, V., Acosta, H., Lopez, S.L., Garrasco, A.E. (2010). Glyphosate-based herbicides promote teratogenic effects on vertebrates by impairing retinoic acid signaling. *Chem Res Toxicol,* Oct 18;23(10):1586-95.

123. Zalecka, A., Bugel, S., Paoletti, F., Kahl, J., Bonanno, A. (2014). The influence of organic production on food quality research findings, gaps and future challenges. *J Sci Food Agric,* Oct;94;(13):2600-4.

124. Ibid. Zalecka. (2014).

125. Mitchell, A.E., Hong, Y.J., Barrett, D.M., Bryant, D.E., Denison, R.F., et al. (2007). Ten-Year Comparison of the Influence of Organic and Conventional Crop Management Practices on the Content of Flavonoids in Tomatoes. *J Agric Food Chem,* Jul 25;55(15):6154-9.

126. Hallmann, E., Lipowski, J., Marszalek, K., Rembialkowska, E. (2013). The seasonal variation in bioactive compounds content in juice from organic and nonorganic tomatoes. *Plant Foods Hum Nutr,* Jun;68(2):171-6.

127. Palupi, E., Jayanegara, A., Ploeger, A., Kahl, J. (2012). Comparison of nutritional quality between conventional and organic dairy products: a meta-analysis. *J Sci Food Agric,* Nov;92(14):2774-81.

128. Crinnon, W.J. (2010). Organic foods contain higher levels of certain nutrients, lower levels of pesticides, and may provide health benefits for the consumer. *Altern Med Rev,* Apr;15(1):4-12.

129. Reganold, J.P., Wachter, J.M. (2016). Organic agriculture in the twenty-first century. *Nat Plants,* Feb 3;2:15221.

130. Strasser, C., Cavoski, I., Di Cagno, R., Kahl, J., Kesse-Guyot, E., et al. (2015). How the Organic Food System Supports Sustainable Diets and Translates These into Practice. *Front Nutr,* Jun 29;2:19.

131. Clark, W.F., Sontrop, J.M., Huang, S.H., Moist, L., Bouby, N. et al. (2016). Hydration and Chronic Kidney Disease Progression: A Critical Review of the Evidence. *Am J Nephrol,* 43(4):281-92.

132. Guest, J., Grant, R. (2016). Carotenoids and Neurobiological Health. *Adv Neurobiol,* 12:199-228.

133. Whole Grains Council. Grains Compared (chart), Retrieved from https://wholegrainscouncil.org/sites/default/files/thumbnails/image/GrainsComparedAll3.jpg.

134. Bechthold, A., Boeing, H., Schwedhelm, C., Hoffmann, G., Knuppel, S. et al. (2017). Food groups and risk of coronary heart disease, stroke and heart failure: A systematic review and dose-response meta-analysis of prospective studies. *Crit Rev Food Sci Nutr,* Oct 17:0.

135. Elkaim, Y. Food Combining Rules: The Complete Guide. Retrieved from https://yurielkaim.com/food-combining-rules.

136. Morgan, W.A., Clayshulte, B.J. (2000). Pecans lower low-density lipoprotein cholesterol in people with normal lipid levels. *J Am Diet Assoc,* Mar;100(3):312-8.

137. Szalay, J. (2015). Inflammation: Causes, Symptoms & Anti-Inflammatory Diet. *LiveScience.* Retrieved from https://mation.html.

138. Pham-Huy, L.A., He, H., Pham-Huy, C. (2008). Free radicals, antioxidants in disease and health. *Int J Biomed Sci,* Jun; 4(2): 89–96.

139. Chiu, C., Milton, R.C., Gensler, G., Taylor, A. (2007). Association between dietary glycemic index and age-related macular degeneration in nondiabetic participants in the Age-Related Eye Disease Study. *Am J Clin Nutr,* July; (86):180-188.

140. Hitti, M. (2007). High-Sugar Foods May Affect Eyesight. WebMD. Retrieved Apr 18 2018 from https://tion/news/20070713/high-sugar-foods-may-affect-eyesight.

141. Hitti, M. (2005). Healthy Diet May Help Seniors' Vision. WebMD. Retrieved Apr 18 2018 from https://wwwhealth/news/20051227/healthy-diet-may-help-seniors-vision#1.

142. de Munter, JS, Hu FB, Spiegelman D, Franz M, van Dam RM. (2007). Whole grain, bran, and germ intake and risk of type 2 diabetes: a prospective cohort study and systematic review. *PLoS Med,* 4:e261.

143. Beulens, J.W., de Bruijne, L.M., Stolk, R.P, Peeters, P.H., Bots, M.L., et al. (2007). High dietary glycemic load and glycemic index increase risk of

cardiovascular disease among middle-aged women: a population-based follow-up study. *J Am Coll Cardiol*, 50:14-21.

144. Halton, T.L., Willett, W.C., Liu, S., Manson, J.E., Albert, C.M., et al. (2006). Low-carbohydrate-diet score and the risk of coronary heart disease in women. *N Engl J Med*, 355:1991-2002.

145. Anderson, J.W., Randles, K.M., Kendall, C.W., Jenkins, D.J. (2004). Carbohydrate and fiber recommendations for individuals with diabetes: a quantitative assessment and meta-analysis of the evidence. *J Am Coll Nutr*, 23:5-17.

146. Ebbeling, C.B., Leidig, M.M., Feldman, H.A., Lovesky, M.M., Ludwig, D.S. (2007). Effects of a low-glycemic load vs low-fat diet in obese young adults: a randomized trial. *JAMA*, 297:2092-102.

147. Maki, K.C., Rains, T.M., Kaden, V.N., Raneri, K.R., Davidson, M.H. (2007). Effects of a reduced-glycemic-load diet on body weight, body composition, and cardiovascular disease risk markers in overweight and obese adults. *Am J Clin Nutr*, 85:724-34.

148. WebMD. How to Use the Glycemic Index. Retrieved May 30 2018 from https://carbs#1.

149. Buyken, A.E., Goletzke, J., Joslowski, G., Felbick, A., Cheng, G., et al. (2014). Association between carbohydrate quality and inflammatory markers: systematic review of observational and interventional studies. *Am J Clin Nutr*, 99(4): 2014;813-33.

150. Ibid. WebMD. How to Use the Glycemic Index.

151. Doheny, K. (2012). Americans Sweet on Sugar: Time to Regulate? WebMD. Retrieved from https://sweet-on-sugar-time-to-regulate#1.

152. Chiu, C., Milton, R.C., Gensler, G., Taylor, A. (2007). Association between dietary glycemic index and age-related macular degeneration in nondiabetic participants in the Age-Related Eye Disease Study. *Am J Clin Nutr*, July; (86):180-188.

153. Hitti, M. (2005). Healthy Diet May Help Senior's Vision. WebMD. Retrieved Apr 18 2018 from https://wwwhealth/news/20051227/healthy-diet-may-help-seniors-vision#1.

154. Hitti, M. (2007). High-Sugar Foods May Affect Eyesight. WebMD. Retrieved Apr 18 2018 from https://wwwtion/news/20070713/high-sugar-foods-may-affect-eyesight.

155. Johnson, R.J., Nakagawa, T., Sanchez-Lozada, L.G., Shafiu, M., Sundaram, S., et al. (2013). Sugar, uric acid, and the etiology of diabetes and obesity. *Diabetes*, Oct;62(10):3307-15.

156. Ibid. WebMD. Food Additives.

157. Hyman, M. (2011). *5 Reasons High Fructose Corn Syrup Will Kill You*. Retrieved from http://drhyman.com/blog/2011/05/13/5-reasons-high-fructose-corn-syrup-will-kill-you.

158. Legeza, B., Marcolongo, P., Gamberucci, A., Varga, V., Banhegyi, G. (2017). Fructose, Glucocorticoids and Adipose Tissue: Implications for the Metabolic Syndrome. *Nutrients*, Apr. 26;9(5).

159. Noble, E.E., Hsu, T.M., Liang, J., Kanoski, S.E. (2017). Early-life sugar consumption has long-term negative effects on memory function in male rats. *Nutr Neurosci*, Sept 25:1-11.

160. Mozaffarian, D., Katan, M.B., Ascherio, A., Stampfer, M.J., Willett, W.C. (2006). Trans fatty acids and cardiovascular disease. *N Engl J Med*, Apr 13; 354(15):1601-13.

161. Cahill, L.E., Pan, A., Chiuve, S.E., Sun, Q., Willett, W.C., et al. (2014). Friedfood consumption and risk of type 2 diabetes and coronary artery disease: a prospective study in 2 cohorts of US women and men. *Am J Clin Nutr*, Aug;100(2):667-675.

162. Association of Food and Drug Officials. Food Color Additives Banned in the USA. Retrieved from banned-in-the-usa.html.

163. Seattle Organic Restaurants. Top 10 foods, additives and preservatives that are banned in many countries except US. Retrieved from http://www.seattleorganicrestaurants.com/vegan-whole-food/foods-banned-in-other-countriesbut-we-eat-in-us.php.

164. Bjarnadottir, A. (2015). How to Read Food Labels Without Being Tricked. Healthline Newsletter. Retrieved from https://tion/how-to-read-food-labels#section3.

165. WebMD. Food Additives: What's Hiding in Your Food? (2017). Retrieved from https://ditives-infographic.

166. Ibid. WebMD. Food Additives.

167. Ritz, E., Hahn, K., Ketteler, M., Kuhlmann, M.K., Mann, J. (2012). Phosphate Additives in Food--A Health Risk. *Dtsch Arztebl Int*, Jan;109(4):49–55.

168. Thiamine. Wikipedia. Retrieved from https://en.wikipedia.org/wiki/Thiamine.

169. Ibid. WebMD. Food Additives.

170. Ibid. WebMD. Food Additives.

171. Gokcen, B.B., Sanlier, N. (2017). Coffee Consumption and Disease Correlations. *Crit Rev Food Sci Nutr*, Aug 30:1-13.

172. Pasquale, L.R., Wiggs, J.L., Willett, W.C., Kang, J.H. (2012). The Relationship between Caffeine and Coffee Consumption and Exfoliation Glaucoma or Glaucoma Suspect: A Prospective Study in Two Cohorts. *Invest Ophthalmol Vis Sci*, Sept. Vol.53, 6427-6433.

173. Nieber, K. (2017). The Impact of Coffee on Health. *Planta Med*, Jul 4.

174. Gulland, A. (2017). Scientists wake up to coffee's benefits. *BMJ*, Nov 22;359:j5381.

175. Brooks, P.J., Zakhari, S. (2013). Moderate alcohol consumption and breast cancer in women: from epidemiology to mechanisms and interventions. *Alcohol Clin Exp Res*, Jan;37(1):23-30.

177. Freeman, D. 12 Health Risks of Chronic Heavy Drinking. Retrieved April 18 2018 from https://wwwhealth-risks-of-chronic-heavy-drinking#1.

178. Lieber, C.S. (2003). Relationship between nutrition, alcohol use, and liver disease. *Alcohol Res Health*, 37(3):220-31.

179. Ibid. Lieber. (2003).

About the Authors

Marc Grossman, OD, LAc, is a doctor of optometry and a licensed acupuncturist. For well over four decades, he has helped many people to maintain healthy vision and even improve their eyesight. He is best described as a holistic eye doctor, dedicated to helping people with conditions ranging from myopia and dry eye to potentially vision-threatening diseases such as macular degeneration and glaucoma. His multidisciplinary approach, which combines nutrition, eye exercises, lifestyle changes, and traditional Chinese medicine, provides him with a wide array of tools to tackle difficult eye problems.

Dr. Grossman is the author of the internationally best-selling book *Magic Eye Beyond 3D: Improve Your Vision* and *Greater Vision: A Comprehensive Program for Physical, Emotional and Spiritual Clarity,* and a coauthor of *Natural Eye Care: A Comprehensive Manual for Practitioners of Oriental Medicine* and *Natural Eye Care: Your Guide to Healthy Vision & Healing.*

Michael Edson, LAc, received his master's degree from Stony Brook University. In addition, he holds a master's degree in Chinese Medicine and is a licensed acupuncturist and certified herbalist. He is a coauthor of *Natural Eye Care: A Comprehensive Manual for Practitioners of Oriental Medicine* and the author of *Natural Brain Support: Your Guide to Preventing and Treating Alzheimer's, Dementia and Other Related Diseases Naturally.* He is a cofounder and the president of Natural Eye Care, Inc., and lives in Yonkers, New York.

Index

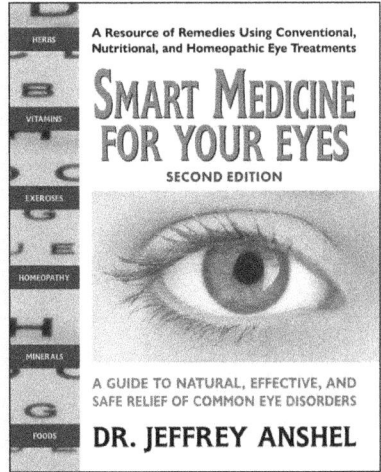

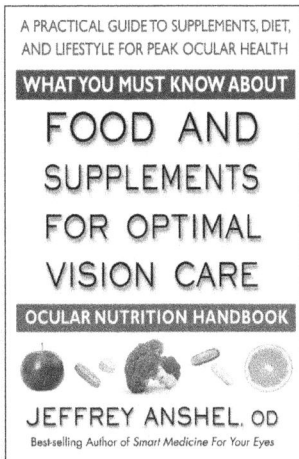

What You Must Know About Dry Eye

How to Prevent, Stop, or Reverse Dry Eye Disease

Jeffrey Anshel, OD

Dry eye can result in eye fatigue, blurred vision, discomfort, and pain. *What You Must Know About Dry Eye* explains the causes of this condition, and then provides a range of treatments—from over-the-counter artificial tears to a proven supplement plan for providing relief.

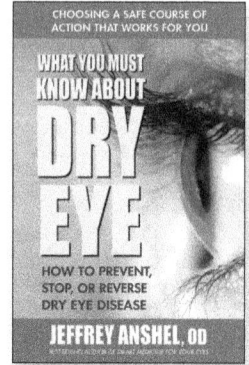

$16.95 • 144 pages • 6 x 9-inch paperback • ISBN 978-0-7570-0479-7

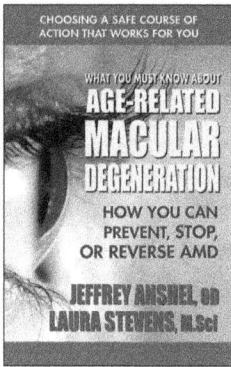

What You Must Know About Age-Related Macular Degeneration

How You Can Prevent, Stop, or Reverse AMD

Jeffrey Anshel, OD, and Laura Stevens, M.Sci

Based on current research, *What You Must Know About Age-Related Macular Degeneration* is a comprehensive guide to preventing, treating, and even reversing age-related macular degeneration through nutritional supplements, the Anti-AMD Diet, and simple lifestyle changes.

$17.95 • 288 pages • 6 x 9-inch paperback • ISBN 978-0-7570-0449-0

What You Must Know About Eyestrain

Jeffrey Anshel, OD

Do you often rub your eyes, experience headaches, or have problems focusing your vision? If so, you may be suffering from eyestrain. *What You Must Know About Eyestrain* provides you with the up-to-date information required to identify the source of the problem and protect your precious vision.

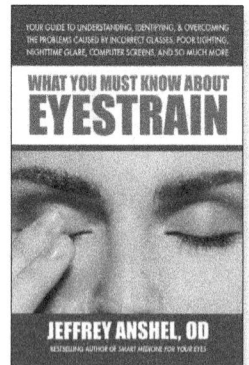

$16.95 • 192 pages • 6 x 9-inch paperback • 978-0-7570-0501-5